Practic
Cardio

Disclaimer

Notice

The author has used his best efforts to provide information that is up-to-date and accurate and is generally accepted within medical standards at the time of publication. However, as the medical science is constantly changing and human error is always possible, neither the author nor the others involved with the publication of this book warrant that the information presented here are absolutely accurate or complete, nor they are responsible for omissions or errors in this book or for the results of using this information. Readers are advised to confirm the information contained in this book with other sources.

Practical Cardiotocography

Third Edition

AK Debdas MD (Kol) FRCOG (Lond) FRCS (Edin) FICOG

Honorary Associate Professor
MGM Medical College, Jamshedpur

Visiting Consultant
Tinplate Hospital, Jamshedpur

Chairman
Indian College of Obstetrics and Gynaecology

Ex-Chairman
Practical Obstetrics Committee, FOGSI

Member
Journal Committee, FOGSI

Peer Reviewer
International Journal of Obstetrics and Gynaecology
British Journal of Obstetrics & Gynaecology

Member
Representative Committee
Royal College of Obstetricians and
Gynaecologists of London - 4 terms

Past President
Indian Society of Perinatology and Reproductive Biology

Past Vice-President
FOGSI

JAYPEE BROTHERS MEDICAL PUBLISHERS (P) LTD

New Delhi • London • Philadelphia • Panama

Jaypee Brothers Medical Publishers (P) Ltd

Headquarters

Jaypee Brothers Medical Publishers (P) Ltd
4838/24, Ansari Road, Daryaganj
New Delhi 110 002, India
Phone: +91-11-43574357
Fax: +91-11-43574314
Email: jaypee@jaypeebrothers.com

Overseas Offices

J.P. Medical Ltd
83 Victoria Street, London
SW1H 0HW (UK)
Phone: +44-2031708910
Fax: +02-03-0086180
Email: info@jpmedpub.com

Jaypee-Highlights Medical Publishers Inc.
City of Knowledge, Bld. 237, Clayton
Panama City, Panama
Phone: +507-301-0496
Fax: +507-301-0499
Email: cservice@jphmedical.com

Jaypee Brothers Medical Publishers Ltd
The Bourse
111 South Independence Mall East
Suite 835, Philadelphia, PA 19106, USA
Phone: + 267-519-9789
Email: ljoe.rusko@jaypeebrothers.com

Jaypee Brothers Medical
Publishers (P) Ltd
Shorakhute, Kathmandu
Nepal
Phone: +00977-9841528578
Email: jaypee.nepal@gmail.com

Jaypee Brothers Medical Publishers (P) Ltd
17/1-B Babar Road, Block-B, Shaymali
Mohammadpur, Dhaka-1207
Bangladesh
Mobile: +08801912003485
Email: jaypeedhaka@gmail.com

Website: www.jaypeebrothers.com
Website: www.jaypeedigital.com

© 2013, AK Debdas

Inquiries for bulk sales may be solicited at: jaypee@jaypeebrothers.com

This book has been published in good faith that the contents provided by the author contained herein are original, and is intended for educational purposes only. While every effort is made to ensure accuracy of information, the publisher and the author specifically disclaim any damage, liability, or loss incurred, directly or indirectly, from the use or application of any of the contents of this work. If not specifically stated, all figures and tables are courtesy of the author. Where appropriate, the readers should consult with a specialist or contact the manufacturer of the drug or device.

Practical Cardiotocography
First Edition: 1998
Second Edition: 2005
Reprint 2008
Third Edition: **2013**

ISBN 978-93-5090-356-8

Printed at Rajkamal Electric Press, Plot No. 2, Phase-IV, Kundli, Haryana.

To
All women
Who must undertake
This serious responsibility
For the mankind

To
The "Princess"

Preface to the Third Edition

This is what the FIGO President Prof S Arulkumaran said recently about CTG: "Until a perfect method is devised to detect intrapartum hypoxia, the importance of the judicious use and meticulous interpretation of the CTG will continue to dominate the science of fetal surveillance (D'Souza and Arulkumaran, 2009)". Here is to add two future 'mantras' (charm words) to it:

greater specificity and total non-invasiveness.

Yes, several new devices are under trial which can pick-up excellent F-ECG from the maternal abdominal surface which would subserve both the above objectives. As regards to toco part of the monitor also, introduction of the completely external multi-parameter technique called uterine electromyography, which records the electrical activity of the uterine muscle, is expected to replace the present highly invasive intrauterine catheter technique.

Golden days for CTG are round the corner!

AK Debdas

Jamshedpur
January 2013

Preface to the First Edition

Cardiotocography is here to stay for the foreseeable future (Carter and Steer, 1993) if not for its positive benefit but certainly for want of a better and simpler method than this of fetal monitoring. Past 25 years have seen phenomenal growth of its user especially in developed countries—the machine now features even in the private chambers of single-handed Obstetricians.

Serial NSTs for high-risk antenatal cases and those with diminished fetal movement is really the bare minimum objective antenatal fetal care that one can give today. As regards to fetal care in labour, a quick FAST with CTG on admission in labour to sort out which fetus should be monitored clinically, which electronically (by CTG), which continuously, which intermittently and which should be taken up straight for caesarean section is gradually coming in vogue. And hence, the pressing need for the obstetric staff—both doctors and midwives to be thoroughly conversant with this investigative technique.

The book is directed to the current user to help him or her to use the machine to the fullest and finest extent and to the prospective user to help to clear his or her doubt about the technique and interpretation and also to help one make the right choice of machine for one's particular requirement. For postgraduate students, it is a must for strengthening their foundation and stimulating their imagination and ingenuity.

I have tried to incorporate in this book my experience of this method since 1971, initially in UK and last 15 years in Telco Maternity Hospital at Jamshedpur, India where I have been training doctors and midwives in this technique for Indian College of Maternity and Child Health.

AK Debdas

1st January, 1998

Acknowledgments

This is not enough acknowledgment to just mention the name – Dr Mrs Rajkumari Debdas (my wife) – for the all-round help that I received from her at every step in preparation of this book right from its first edition and through its three editions.

Of course, to Shri Jitendar P Vij (Group Chairman) Jaypee Brothers Medical Publishers (P) Ltd. I am extremely grateful for being with me since the nineties when the use of CTG in India was very rare. I must express that it is a great service on his part to take upon himself to make this 'made easy' volume of a very complex technology available to the specialists at large in India.

This book—*Practical Cardiotocography*—is almost synonymous with CTG workshops in India and thanks to the Organisers of these workshops for their appreciation of this work.

Acknowledgments

Contents

Plate 1

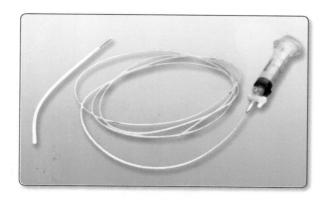

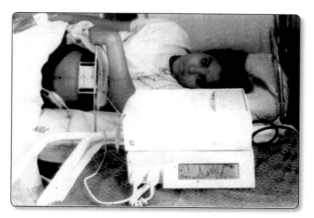

Cardiotocography in action

Plate 2

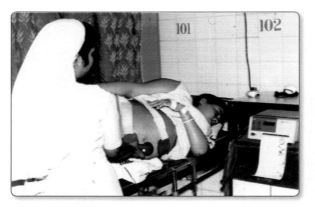

Vibroacoustic stimulation being given

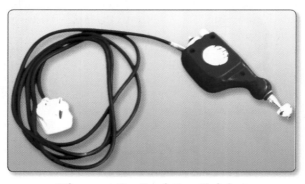

Vibroacoustic stimulation (Debdas)

What is Cardiotocography

Cardiotocography (CTG) is a procedure of graphically (graphy) recording fetal heart activity (cardio) and uterine contraction (toco)—both recorded in the same time scale simultaneously and continuously through uterine quiescence and contraction.

Though originally designed to monitor the fetus during labor so as to see how it performed on the face of the circulatory stress brought about by uterine contraction (see later), the scope of the method has now been widely enlarged to include the antenatal period as well where uterine contraction is not a factor except when it is artificially generated just for the test as in contraction stress test. (Caldeyro-Barcia and Alvarez, 1952; Hon EH, 1959; Cunningham et al, 2001).

It may be interesting to note that over the years CTG has become synonymous with the term 'fetal monitoring' and the CTG machine has come to be referred as the 'Fetal Monitor', and this is no wonder because 85% of births in USA get monitored by CTG (National Vital Statistics Report, USA, 2003).

FURTHER READING

1. Caldeyro-Barcia, R Alvarez HJ. Obstet Gynaec Brit Emp 1952;59:646.
2. Hon EH. Obstet Gynec 1959;14:154.
3. National Vital Statistics Report, USA, 2003
4. William's Obstetrics: 23rd Edition, Edited by Cunningham FG, Leveno KJ, Bloom SL, et al. Intrapartum Assessment, Mc Graw Hill, New York, 2010;410-43.

CHAPTER 2

Pioneers of Cardiotocography

Cardiotocography, a revolutionary method of fetal monitoring, was first introduced in late 1950s. The main credit for it goes to the following two great obstetricians—Professor EH Hon of Southern California and Professor R Cladeyro Barcia of Uruguay.

The other two pioneers in this field are Professor GS Daws and Professor C. Redman of United Kingdom who, in the eighties, gave a large leap to the procedure by developing a CTG analysis algorithm and devising a computer programme based on it for on-line, uniform, ultraprecise analysis and reporting of the graph.

Credit must also go to Professor R W Beard and his team of United Kingdom for producing for the first time the hard evidence that — even with the worst pattern of CTG tracing only 50–60 percent of fetuses were acidotic which shook up the whole speciality.

Credit should also go to Professor Karl G Rosen of Sweden who, with the endeavor of curing the above deficiency of the CTG monitoring, succeeded in incorporating fetal electrocardiography (ECG) as an integral part of CTG. His noteworthy contribution was addition of an in-built STAN software (ST analyzer) which can instantly on line analyse the pathological CTG tracing as to whether it was causing myocardial ischemia in the fetus or not without having to resort to an additional invasive procedure like Fetal Blood Sampling. Obviously, this is a major quality and convenience dimension to the CTG procedure.

FURTHER READING

1. Beard RW, Filshie GM, Knight CA, et al. The significance of the changes in the continuous fetal heart rate in the first stage of labor. Obstet Gynaecol Br C Wlth 1971;78:865-81.
2. Caldeyro-Barcia R, Alvarez H, Reynolds SRM. Surg Gynec Obstet 1950; 91:641.
3. Dawes G, Lobb M, Moulden M, et al. Antenatal cardiotocogram quality and interpretation using computers. Brit J Obstet Gynaecol 1992;99:791-97.
4. Hon EH. Amer J Obstet Gynec 1959;77:1084.
5. Laybourne M, Mander AM. The role of computerized antenatal fetal heart rate analysis in obstetric practice. In: John Studd (Ed). Progress in Obstetrics and Gynaecology. London: Churchill Livingstone. 2000;14:188-201.
6. Rosen KG, Kjellmer I. Changes in fetal heart rate and ECG during hypoxia. Acta Physiol Scand 1975;93:59-66.

Scope of Use of Cardiotocography

ANTENATALLY

1. Cardiotocography (CTG) can accurately and continuously assess the baseline fetal heart (FH) behavior including its baseline variability, i.e. the critical beat to beat variation of its baseline rate. This later parameter which provides vital information about the fetal oxygen status is not assessable by clinical means.

2. It can precisely (quantitatively) assess FH response to fetal movement.

3. It can assess fetal heart (FH) behaviour in response to Braxton–Hicks contraction.

4. It can objectively double check the fetal movement count by the mother specially when her counting is low or when she can't feel any movement at all or she is unsure about it (Acto-cardiography).

5. It can check the movement profile of the fetus which, it has been assumed, should be able to assess its general physical state and may be its behaviour pattern and through that the integrity of its central nervous system. Movement profile also logically should give some idea about the nutritional state/energy balance of the fetus because growth retarded and chronically ill fetus is expected to move less.

6. It can provisionally diagnose intrauterine death by proving the absence of fetal heart beat.

7. It provides objective help in the diagnosis of "false pain" by its ability of objectively recording the occurrence or otherwise of 'true' uterine contractions

8. It can objectively diagnose or exclude premature onset of labor and can judge the effect of tocolytic therapy on a diagnosed case. It is, in fact, necessary for titration of the dose of tocolytics. The latest in this area is home and ambulatory uterine activity (irritability) monitoring in susceptible cases. Points 7 and 8 are purely toco function

9. It can serially, though indirectly, monitor fetal oxygen status and hence is indispensable for monitoring intra-uterine growth retardation (IUGR), post-dated pregnancy, pregnant diabetics, etc.

10. Fetal vibroacoustic stimulation test (VAST) automatically tests fetal hearing in addition to assessing its oxygen status.

11. Application of VAST reduces the false positively rate of conventional nonstressed CTG (NST-see later) by 50 percent while at the same time reducing the duration of CTG monitoring to half.

12. Some of the drugs given to the mother like sedatives, anticonvulsants, drugs acting on sympatho-adrenal system, etc. (used in the treatment of hypertensive disorders in pregnancy) can affect both fetal movement and fetal heart rate pattern. CTG can indirectly assess the effects of these drugs on the fetus.

13. CTG provides objective non-invasive monitoring of twins even during antenatal period which is *impossible* clinically.

14. As quoted widely in the literature, *the main role of antenatal CTG is to allow more woman with high-risk pregnancy to continue their pregnancy to greater maturity, safer maturity, better inducibility or until spontaneous onset of labor.*

INTRANATALY

1. The foremost use of CTG during labor is to diagnose fetal distress "early" i.e. before the occurrence of gross acidosis and before hypoxic brain damage.

2. CTG by exhibiting typical tracing pattern can *diagnose cord compression* specially occult cord compression and/or cord overstretching if that happens to occur with uterine contraction during labor.

3. CTG by its tocometry facility can convincingly diagnose abnormal uterine contraction specially *hypotonic inertia and hypertonus* which are **not** possible to diagnose by clinical means.

4. Only under the CTG guidance one is able to use oxytocin stimulation in patients with relatively higher risk of rupture of uterus, e.g. in a post-cesarean case, in a grand multipara, etc. by accurately monitoring the amplitude of changes in intra-amniotic fluid pressure caused by contraction.

5. CTG also provides objective monitoring of *twins* during labor which is **not** possible clinically.

6. CTG can indirectly diagnose *head compression* during labor by exhibiting typical trace pattern – Type I Dip (see later).

7. *'Admission test'* – This is a very useful application of CTG in labor. By this it is possible to determine the monitoring requirement of an individual fetus right at the beginning of labour like -
   a. Whether a fetus needs just clinical monitoring or
   b. It needs more precise CTG monitoring.
   c. Whether it needs continuous CTG monitoring or
   d. Intermittent CTG monitoring.

   Besides, it also, by the characters and gravity of the tracing, can indicate which patient (fetus) should not be allowed to proceed in labor (i.e. those which will be found to show CTG signs of compromise even right at the beginnig of labor) and in which it is safe for the labor to proceed.

8. For the cases showing abnormal tracing during the course of labor the necessity for fetal blood sampling (for detection of fetal acidosis) can be reduced by 50 percent by employment of fetal vibroacoustic stimulation to the conventional CTG procedure (see Chapter 19).

9. Fetal ECG can be obtained with the help of scalp electrode of CTG which can be used to diagnose fetal myocardial ischemia (see Chapter 21)

10. CTG is a must to cover labor of *high-risk cases.*

11. CTG is a must to cover labor of thin *meconium cases.* The need of CTG monitoring, of course, is most urgent in thick meconium cases but thick meconium cases should be dealt with like an emergency.

12. CTG is a necessity for doing *augmentation of labor* specially to avoid Hyperstimulation and its consequent fetal and maternal hazard.

13. CTG is a necessity for covering fetal risks of *epidural analgesia*

14. CTG is a necessity to monitor laboring mothers having pyrexia (Edwin and Arulkumaran, 2008)

15. CTG is a highly logical and kind solution to the undeniable human factors/human lapses of manual fetal monitoring of labor—the event being necessarily a very prolonged (12–18 hours) and taxing affair even for care giver.

FURTHER READING

1. Cunningham FG, Leveno KJ, Bloom SL, et al. In William's Obstetrics, 23rd Edition, Intrapartum Assessment, Mc Graw Hill, New York, 2010;410-43.

2. Edwin C, Arulkumaran S: Electronic Fetal Heart Monitoring in current & future practice, The Journal of O & G of India, Vol 58, 2008;121-30.

3. Myles Textbook for Midwives:Edited by Fraser DM and Cooper MA, Monitoring the Fetus, Church Livingstone, London, 15th Edition, 2009;481-84.

The Need for Cardiotocographic Monitoring

- Technical need
- Physiological need
- The Social need
- Professional need
- Need from Manpower angle
- The Medico-legal need

THE TECHNICAL NEED
During Antenatal Period

- Macerated stillbirth still constitutes a major cause of perinatal mortality
- The process of antenatal fetal demise is silent, i.e. it is symptomless and often even signless
- The predictability of clinical methods of antenatal fetal monitoring is poor
- Though fetal movement (FM) count by the mother is a good screening test for fetal well-being – its reliability is low in the very cases where it needs to be the highest, i.e. in the cases when the count is low. So any action taken just on low FM count without CTG verification is likely to be grossly wrong.
- When one has to solely depend on clinical monitoring, specially in high-risk cases it is often associated with unaccountable high

rate of unnecessary panic induction then failed induction and cesarean section leading to high cost and high morbidity. Objective monitoring by CTG can reduce this number.

During Intranatal Period

Though intranatal period is more amenable to clinical monitoring (period to be monitored being limited)—it has three significant problems:

a. Impracticability of monitoring fetal heart clinically during uterine contraction, i.e. at the most stressful phase for the fetus when it needs the most critical monitoring (see below).

b. Impracticability of precisely monitoring the stresser, i.e. the uterine contraction clinically—specially its basal tone (hypertonus) and amplitude.

c. Impracticability of arranging *one to one manning* for all labor cases for effective clinical monitoring. However, it must be appreciated that clinical monitoring with one to one manning would be *far more expensive than CTG* monitoring because this would need a very large number of Nurses.

CTG can overcome all above problem.

PHYSIOLOGICAL NEED

This applies to intranatal period only.

The *uterine contractions* of labor act as 'living ligature' for the feeding vessels to the placenta, i.e. the oxygen channel to the fetus. This makes it mandatory to monitor FH during contractions and soon after that which, as described above, is not very practical clinically confidently.

The other two unique stress factors of labor that work on fetus namely – a) the factor of *head compression* and b) the possible *mechanical cord disturbances* (by its stretching, may be by its compression during uterine contractions) also cannot be monitored clinically.

THE SOCIAL NEED

With changing social milieu, there is now the social pressure of giving 100 percent fetal result every time with every case with allowance for no lapse from whatever source. This is occasioned by the following social changes:

a. Maternity and childbirth today is no longer accepted as the 'be- all' thing by women specially by the educated women. Instead, for a modern woman of today, this overwhelming bio-social event is rather a vitally necessary evil that must be endured to satisfy her *biological ego* and also for being able to have her own unique *biological possession*—her own offspring while at the same time fulfilling her earmarked unique *womanly social responsibility* of perpetuation of her family.

   The reason for viewing maternity so non-emotionally is—this joyous task not only involves a lot of physical discomfort, incapacity, pain and health risk for the woman but it also entails a lot of unfair waste of peak time from her life span during which her male contemporaries overtake her in career. Hence obviously today's women cannot afford to take chances and so also their obstetrician by relying solely and merely on his or her clinical acumen and intelligent guess.

b. There is now the wide acceptance by the community of two children family norm and this must happen as per the individual couple's life plan. Since any derailment of this plan is almost unacceptable by the present day couple hence is the demand on technological assistance like CTG.

c. Everyone in today's society is very pushed for time and has a schedule to meet. So, today the implied social dictum about maternity is "Every mother must do it right the first time and Everytime" and hence, to cater for that, every obstetrician has to use everything that is there in his or her armamentarium to help her to achieve this.

   So, obviously today's obstetrician needs more objective and more precise method of fetal monitoring like CTG, ultrasonography or even better methods.

d. Demand for objectivity. The society today is more educated, more informed, more suspicious. If the obstetrician says that he or she wants to do cesarean for fetal distress – the husband and other relatives want to know: *What evidence do you have for it doctor?*

THE PROFESSIONAL NEED

Intranatal death gives the concerned obstetrician the most horrible feeling of inadequacy, foolishness, guilt and bad name.

CTG by providing proper and timely guidance can help in this regard.

THE NEED FROM MANPOWER ANGLE

CTG can reduce the necessity of requirement of *skilled manpower* in labor room while *improving* the quality and precision of monitoring of both fetus and uterine contraction. It is a major necessity *for busy labor room* with inadequate nursing manning as is almost the rule in developing countries.

THE MEDICO-LEGAL NEED

The newly emerging problem of litigation in medicine, in obstetrics in particular for doing and, more importantly, for not doing in time-calls for some hard evidence of the clinical events on which the obstetrician acted or choose not to act. A CTG tracing constitutes one of such hard evidence.

FURTHER READING

1. Debdas AK. Fetal monitoring by cardiotocography. Indian Journal of Clinical Practice, (IJCP) 1996;69.
2. Debdas AK. Today's ultramodern ways of monitoring fetal well-being, Hindustan Times, 13th October, 1995;11.

3. Magowan B, Owen P, Drife J: Clinical Obst Gynae, 2nd edition, Monitoring the Fetus in labor, Elsevier, Edinburg, pp. 331-43, 2009.

4. Myles Textbook for Midwives:Edited by Fraser DM and Cooper MA, Monitoring the Fetus, Church Livingstone, London, 15th Edition, pp. 481-84, 2009.

5. William's Obstetrics: 23rd Edition, Edited by Cunningham FG, Leveno KJ, Bloom SL, et al. Intrapartum Assessment, Mc Graw Hill, New York, pp. 410-43, 2010.

CHAPTER 5

Methods Used for Picking Up Fetal Heart Activity

Fetal heart activity can be picked up by two methods:
- External method
- Internal method.

EXTERNAL METHOD

Since this method uses 'ultrasound'—this is also called Ultrasound mode. This is the *most commonly* used method.

INTERNAL METHOD

This method uses 'fetal electrocardiography'. Hence, this is also called fetal ECG mode. This method is designed to pick up of the electrical activity of fetal heart 'directly' from the 'fetal body' through placement of electrode on it which is possible only in labor and after rupture of membranes—hence, it is termed the 'internal' method.

This direct fetal ECG mode can be used in two different ways:
- Using it simply for obtaining fetal heart rate (FHR) for conventional internal cardiotocography (CTG)—for which only 'R' wave is brought into operation. All the current internal mode CTG machines uses only this bit of F-ECG (see later)
- Using the full PQRST complex of ECG 'on its own merit'—for predicting the state of oxygenation of the fetus from the analysis

of various characters of the wave-from itself—somewhat like its use in the case of adult (see Chapter 21—"CTG cum fetal ECG— an approach towards precision").

EXTERNAL METHOD OF FETAL HEART (FH) PICK UP
OR

EXTERNAL CARDIOTOCOGRAPHY
(EXTERNAL METHOD OF FETAL MONITORING)

As already mentioned above – this is an Ultrasound (US) mode of FH pick-up.

This method has been presented under the following headings:

- US principle used
- Structure and types of US transducer
- How FHR is computed from echo signal
- Materials required for FH pick up by US mode
- Actual technique of external cardiotocography
- Some operational problems and their solutions
- Drawbacks of external fetal monitoring
- Special advantage of external monitoring.

Principle

This is done by the use of *Doppler Principle* of ultrasound which states that—"frequency of sound wave shifts as the source moves relative to the receiver". Keeping this principle in mind, if one thinks of a beating fetal heart as the source and a Doppler US probe placed over it as the receiver the matter would be immediately clear. In its contracted position the heart is farthest from the probe, whereas in its relaxed position it is nearest to the probe and, hence there is shift in frequency of the ultrasound that echoes back to the probe from the FH compared to the frequency of the original US beam, that was projected towards it from the US probe (US probe is also called US transducer).

The method aims to pick up the 'mechanical activity' of FH (unlike ECG which picks up the electrical activity of FH).

Structure and Types of Ultrasound (US) Transducer

A little knowledge about this is essential in order to understand the mechanism of picking up of FH activity better. Firstly, it should be noted that it is made up of multiple (seven) elements of piezo-electric crystal (**Fig. 5.1**) so that it can emit and receive ultrasound 'over a wide angle' covering some degree of change in fetal (heart) position. Secondly, the elements are so arranged in the transducer that while the central crystal transmits (throws in) the US wave the surrounding six receive its echo. Such transducers emit US 'continuously'. There is, however, another type of transducer which uses 'pulsed' US. In these, the signals are both transmitted and received by the same crystal. The advantage of this system is that—the noise is less and the total amount of sound energy directed to the fetus is also less (Steer, 1986).

US transducer generally operates at a frequency of 1.5 MHz and has a maximum ultrasonic power output density of 4 mW/cm². The machines with antenatal 'dual' fetal monitoring facility for 'twins'

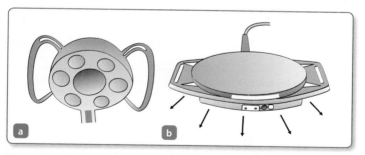

Fig. 5.1 (a) Inside view of maternal surface of an ultrasonic transducer showing seven elements of Piezo-electric crystals. This is not normally visible as it remains covered by a plastic case; (b) Showing the beams of ultrasound coming from the multiple Piezo-electric crystals and covering a wide angle so as to cover the change in fetal position and hence that of its heart

has another additional US transducer usually of 2 MHz frequency with ultrasonic power output density of 12 mW/cm^2 (also see twin monitoring by CTG).

As regards its external structure, its case has been adapted in such a way that it can be easily fixed by a belt on the mother's abdomen. Transducers with a knob on the back to fit in the holes on the belt are much easier to handle than those with brackets on each side (**Fig. 5.2**). Besides the standard type of US transducer as detailed above, some manufacturers make some special types of transducers as described below (**Fig. 5.3**).

'Y' Shaped Transducer

A single main cable goes into the machine. Halfway along it's length the main cable divides into two branch cables at the end of each of which a transducer is attached. To one branch cable is attached US transducer for picking up FH activity and to the other the transducer for recording uterine contraction.

The advantages of this design are two: (i) It is tangle-resistant, so there is no chance of confusion between two transducers or two sockets and (ii) One has to deal with just one socket and one plug, (iii) Chance of cross plugging of FH transducers into toco socket and toco transducer into FH socket is totally avoided. But nowadays, the sockets and the plugs of the two types of the transducers are color matched, e.g. red

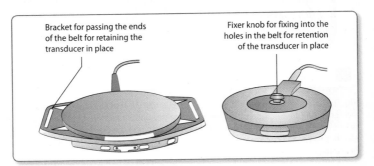

Bracket for passing the ends of the belt for retaining the transducer in place

Fixer knob for fixing into the holes in the belt for retention of the transducer in place

Fig. 5.2 Showing two different arrangements for fixing the transducer to the abdomen by belt

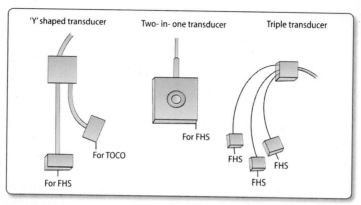

Fig. 5.3 Three special types of transducer

plug goes into the red socket and green plug goes into green socket and thereby the possibility of cross plugging has been removed.

Two-in-One Transducer

A single transducer body contains both US and toco elements. The advantages of this model are that one has to place just one transducer instead of two and the patient has to put up with only one belt rather than two. However, with this combined type, signals cannot be picked up as well as with the use of two separate transducers for two separate functions.

Triple Transducer

This consists of three ultraminiaturised Doppler US transducer. The advantages of this model are:

i. Since a larger area can be monitored with this—fetal rotation during normal labor can be covered without having to re-site the transducer. Descent of the fetus can also be covered by covering the descending location of its heart.

ii. It can additionally monitor fetal movement.

Beltless Transducer

The above triple transducer is so small that it does not require a belt and can be fixed with an adhesive tape alone. The advantage of this design is—*long-term monitoring is possible* with greater patient comfort as in the cases of problematic non-stress test, 'Flat' or straight line CTG traces (see later) which needs prolonged monitoring.

How FHR is Computed from Echo Signal

This is done by measuring the 'time interval' between two consecutive beats (echoes) and then mathematically converting it into beat per minute (BPM). This derived rate is then averaged over 1.2 seconds or for 3 beats. More recently, the BPM is processed with the help of microprocessor using *'autocorrelation technique'* to extract the repetitive FHR (Cunningham et al., 2010). Finally, it is the processed rate that shows up on the FHR display window and on the tracing paper as the beat-to-beat rate. This principle of using 'time interval between beats' to compute the FHR explains the unbelievable ever changing FHR that one sees on the FHR display window—now 140, within a split of a second 144 (BPM) and so on.

Materials Required for FH Pick up by US Mode

(Materials required for external fetal monitoring)
- Ultrasonic transducer
- Aquasonic gel
- Abdominal belt

Ultrasonic Transducer

This has already been described above.

Aquasonic Gel

Since US waves travel very poorly through air and extremely easily through liquids, this gel must be applied in adequate quantity over the entire face of the transducer to eliminate all air between the transducer and the mother's abdomen. In tropical countries like India, as the gel dries up very fast repeated application may be necessary for continued clear pick up of FH activity.

Abdominal Belt

Two types of belts are available: disposable and reusable. Reusable type belts are good enough, but belts with velcro is better avoided because the velcro tends to stick here and there with patients' dress, blanket, etc. 'Tubigrip' (somewhat like lower part of men's vest minus the sleeves) is a suitable alternative for fixing the transducers on mother's abdomen.

Actual Technique of External Cardiotocography

(Only cardio part will be described here—the toco part has been described in Chapter 6)

- Lay the two abdominal belts across the patient's examination table or her bed at about the middle, i.e. the place where the patient's abdomen is likely to be located when she lies on that table or bed. One belt (the lower one) is meant for fixing the US fetal heart transducer and the other belt (the upper belt) is meant for fixing the toco transducer which has to be placed over uterine fundus (see Chapter 6 and also the colored plate No.1 at the beginning of the book). If the patient is already lying on the table, the belt has to be passed under her body to circle around her.
- Patient lies supine after emptying her bladder
- Palpate and auscultate to locate the fetal back and the fetal heart.
- Now plug in the US (cardio) transducer in the appropriate socket of the machine and switch the machine on. As already mentioned, in most machines the US plug and its socket are color matched, i.e. both are of the same color. This is done in order to avoid the possibility of confusing these with those of toco facility, i.e. to avoid cross plugging of two functions.
- Apply a film of aquasonic gel over the entire transducer face and place it over the baby's back. The fetal heart sound (FHS) should be immediately audible. Adjust the volume control to the desired level.

- Now keeping the transducer pressed against the abdominal wall, do a bit of searching of the uterus with it to determine from which of its (transducer's) positions FHS can be heard loudest and clearest. While doing this imagine that a beam of US is going straight in from the face of the transducer (**Fig. 5.4**) and it is this which is doing the searching. Hold the transducer still in the optimally recording position and fix it right on that spot with the help of the belt already laid on the table. Make sure that the belts fit snugly and comfortably.

- With the transducer focussed on the fetal heart, besides the audible FHS, the FHR-as beat per minute (say 140 BPM) should come up on 'digital display' window and the FH flasher light should start flashing (see Chapter 7—General description of CTG machine and **Fig. 7.1**). It is at this stage one should press the 'record switch' to start the rolling of the recording paper. As the paper with FH tracing recorded on, it comes out of the machine note the quality of the tracing.

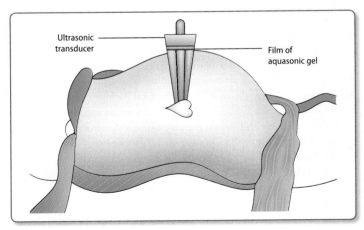

Ultrasonic transducer

Film of aquasonic gel

Fig. 5.4 Fetal heart is under full ultrasound beam of the transducer

- Most models of the CTG machine provide 'signal quality indicator'—green, yellow and red lights—meaning optimal signal, fair signal and unacceptable signal respectively (akin to the significance of the traffic lights). Usually no tracing will be recorded with red light on. This helps in proper positioning of the transducer—right over the fetal heart.

- It is always better to check the mother's pulse to make sure that the transducer is not inadvertently picking up the mother's pulse (aorta). Both the rate and the rhythm of the mother's pulse *should be different* from that of the fetus.

- Once it is all set the patient should be turned to 15° left lateral tilt in order to minimise aortocaval compression.

Some Operational Problems and Their Solutions

Erratic Digital Display

The possible causes of this are—fetal movement, fetal decent, fetal rotation, transducer slip, loosening of the belt and drying up of the gel.

The solution would be—application of a bit more of the gel, relocation of the transducer and tightening of the belt.

Intermittent Dotty Tracing

It's causes and solutions are same as that of the 'erratic digital display' - as given above.

Questionable (very low) Heart Rate

The cause could be that the machine is inadvertently picking the mother's arotic pulsation. Check the mother's pulse to see whether it tallies with the audible FHR. If yes, re-site the transducer over the fetal heart, (see 'doubling' and 'halving' defect later in this chapter).

Too Thick Tracing Line

The cause of this is overheating of the pen tip which should be adjusted by turning the pen heat knob. This happens only with the thermal paper.

Drawbacks of the External Fetal Monitoring

1. It is possible with this mode to inadvertently pick up and monitor the mother's heart rate instead of that of the fetus.
2. The transducer often gets displaced due to maternal movements and needs adjustment.
3. With fetal descent and rotation in labor, the transducer needs resiting.
4. It is not very suitable for FH monitoring in the second stage of labor when bearing down and other uncontrollable excessive maternal movements do not give proper FH tracing during the vital contraction phase.

    None of the above problems exist with internal method which operates by picking up signal 'directly' from the fetal body by means of an electrode placed on it (but internal monitoring is possible only in labor after rupture of membranes).

5. Wearing two abdominal belts for prolonged period is uncomfortable, more so in hot countries.
6. The patient remains tied to the machine, hence it is physically very restricting. This problem is also there with the internal method of monitoring. The solution to this is 'telemetry' (see Chapter 28) which is somewhat more expensive.
7. The parameter of beat-to-beat variation is not as precise with this method as it is with the internal (direct ECG) method.
8. Very rarely the rate becomes halved or doubled or it changes abruptly by more than 35 bpm. While in most cases, the event being so odd, one attends to the machine rather than the fetus. However, in rare instances these may be interpreted as true acceleration or deceleration. This error is more likely to occur when the true FHR drops below 90 bpm, or rises above 200 bpm as explained below.

Mechanism of 'Doubling'

When the FHR drops to approximately 90 bpm or less , heart movements gradually become so far apart that it is possible for ultrasonic monitors to interpret, "two heart movements belonging to a single beat"—as two separate heart beats. This produces an FHR tracing that is double the actual heart rate. This is called 'doubling' defect.

Mechanism of 'Halving'

When the FHR increases to 200 bpm or greater, heart movements gradually become close together. In this situation ultrasonic transducers may interpret two separate heart beats as a single beat and produces a tracing of half the actual rate by half-counting the real rate.

Hence sudden 'counter' changes in baseline, e.g. large jump in heart rate during severe bradycardia or sudden drop in baseline rate during severe tachycardia should be interpreted very carefully. In such situations, it is best to recheck FHR by fetoscope.

Special Advantages of the External Monitoring

1. External monitoring is non-invasive.
2. Very little skill is required for its application. Can be done by a nurse.
3. It is more agreeable for the patient because vaginal manipulation is not involved.
4. It can be used both for antenatal and also for intranatal fetal monitoring. In fact, the external method can be used right from the 16th week of gestation. In comparison the internal method cannot be used at all for antenatal monitoring because it needs direct access to the fetal body.
5. It is less expensive, i.e. there is no recurring expense of buying the electrode unlike that for internal monitoring.
6. There is no chance of injury to the fetus or the mother.
7. It does not interfere with vaginal examination during labor. (In the internal method one has to be very careful during vaginal examination because with this there remains the chance of causing dislocation of the scalp electrode during the process).

INTERNAL METHOD OF FH SIGNAL PICK UP

OR

INTERNAL CARDIOTOCOGRAPHY (INTERNAL FETAL MONITORING)

As already mentioned, this is an ECG mode of FH pick up. This has been presented below under the following headings:

- Physical principle
- Structure and types of fetal ECG electrode
- The electrode applicator
- How FHR is computed from fetal ECG
- Materials required for internal CTG
- Actual technique of doing internal CTG
- Some operational problems and their solutions
- Drawbacks of internal fetal monitoring
- Special advantage of internal monitoring

Physical Principle

Internal cardiotocography is accomplished by obtaining a 'direct fetal ECG' by picking up the electrical activity of FH directly from the fetal body through placement of electrode on it. Hence the internal method can only be applied during labor with a minimum of 2 cm dilatation of the cervix and ruptured membranes.

Structure and Types of Fetal ECG Electrode

This has four components—a metal hook, a small plastic body, two long thin wires usually one red and one white, entwined with each other and, fourthly, bits of wax at the ends of these wires to seal them off (**Fig. 5.5**).

The purpose of the *hook* are two: (a) to penetrate and anchor the electrode on the skin of the presenting part of the fetus and (b) to act as one of the electrical poles of ECG. Some models have two hooks,

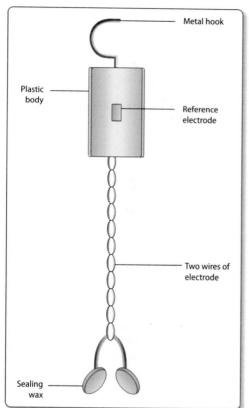

Fig. 5.5 Structure of fetal (Spiral) electrode

some models have one hook and some have a clip (like Mitchel's clip) instead of hook. Those with hook are also called 'spiral electrodes' or 'screw electrodes' because they look somewhat like a spiral and have to be screwed in place (**Fig. 5.6**). These are also called 'scalp electrode' because they are most often placed on fetal scalp.

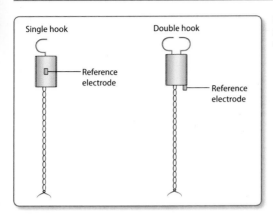

Fig. 5.6 Showing two types fetal electrode

Two other types of electrode are also available—namely: "Safety Slip" electrode (which does not get overturned) and "surgicraft Copeland" type electrode (easier placement).

The *plastic body* incorporates the second pole of ECG which can be seen as two exposed metallic points on its surface or base (**Fig. 5.6**) known as vaginal 'reference electrode'.

This bit of design is most ingenious in that the second pole makes contact with the mother's body through the electrolyte content of her own cervical and vaginal secretion present locally—the *Saline Electrical Bridge* (Cunningham et al., 2010). This clever design can do away with the necessity of placement of an additional thigh electrode (maternal) for recording fetal ECG. But this external Reference electrode on the maternal thigh helps to element the electrical interference. In doing fetal ECG, the electrical potential of the fetal electrode is compared with that of the vaginal reference electrode.

The wax seal at the end of the wires must be removed before making connection.

The electrode wires are to be connected to the 'connector cable' through its 'clamp block' (**Fig. 5.7**).

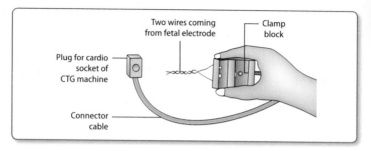

Fig. 5.7 Connector cable with clamp block. The two wires coming from fetal electrode are clamped in the clamp block. Electrical signal coming from the fetus is then carried to the CTG machine through the connector cable which is to be plugged into the cardio socket of CTG machine

The Electrode Applicator

The 'fetal electrode set' as described above comes in a ready-to-use sterilised disposable pack housed in its applicator the design of which varies from manufacturer to manufacturer.

How FHR is Computed from Fetal ECG

Fetal ECG, as it is being recorded, is fed continuously into a cardio-tachometer and the machine is so designed that only 'R' waves can trigger the tachometer. The machine automatically and continuously measures the R-R interval (**Fig. 5.8**) and then mathematically works out the FHR—as beat per minute (BPM) from this 'R-R interval'—just as it is done from the 'echo interval' in the case of external monitoring by US mode (as already described).

Materials Required for Internal Cardiotocography

- Spiral Electrode (Fetal electrode)
- Connector Cable Set
- Thigh Belt

Spiral Electrode

This has already been described above.

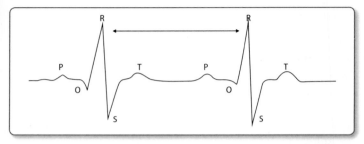

Fig. 5.8 ECG tracing showing R-R interval. It is the 'R' which is used to trigger the cardiotocograph and the R-R interval is used to compute the FHR and beat to beat variability

Connector Cable Set (Fig. 5.7)

This has a clamp block and a cable with a plug at the end of the cable. The clamp block is meant for taking the 2 wires coming from the spiral electrode and any of the two wires can be fitted into any of the two holes of the clamp—the polarity is automatically corrected by the machine. The clamp block has to be belted over the right upper thigh of the 'mother' with the help of 'thigh belt' provided.

The cable plug has to be plugged into the machine in the appropriate socket, usually, marked as 'cardio' socket or 'Direct ECG' socket. Once this connection is made the fetus gets connected to the machine.

Thigh Belt

This is meant for fixing the connector cable-set to the mothers' upper thigh (**Fig. 5.10**).

Actual Technique of doing Internal CTG

a.   Application of Scalp Electrode
b.   Electrical Connection
c.   Operation of the CTG Machine
d.   When to remove the electrode
e.   How to remove the electrode
f.   How to record fetal arrhythmia

Procedure of Application of Scalp Electrode

- Patient is placed in lithotomy position.
- A vaginal examination is done under usual aseptic precaution to ascertain that the requisite conditions for application are satisfied, i.e. cervical dilation of at least 2 cm and the station of the presenting part within 2 cm from ischial spines.
- The electrode set in its applicator is then introduced into the vagina under the guidance of the vaginal finger and positioned 'at right angle' to the presenting part. Do ENSURE that (a) the electrode is not placed on any of the fontanelle, (b) never on baby's face or (c) on it's genitalia (in case of breech presentation). As a general rule, spiral electrodes are fixed on the fetal body by 'clockwise' rotation (**Fig. 5.9**).
- The actual technique of application of the electrode varies with the make and model of the electrode and its particular applicator but

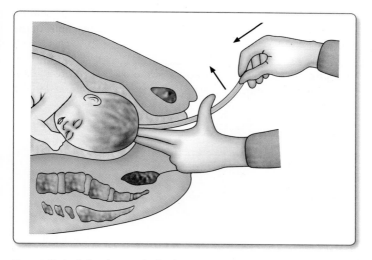

Fig. 5.9 Method of application of scalp electrode—it is applied by turning the applicator in clockwise direction after steadying it in place perpendicular to the head while the two vaginal fingers guide and support the applicator

the procedure is not at all difficult—only it needs a little practice. It is best to practice the manuovre of delivering and anchoring the electrode first on a stretched glove skin outside the body before trying it on a fetus.

Electrical Connection

• The machine is to be plugged into the mains through a 3 pin plug with earthing as usual.

• The plug of the 'Connector Cable' (**Fig. 5.7**) is next plugged into the socket on the CTG machine labelled as either 'Cardio' or 'Direct ECG'.

• Next, as the patient lies in lithotomy position, an assistant ties the 'thigh belt' (**Fig. 5.10**) around her right upper thigh (right—because the machine is usually placed on the patient's right side).

• The 'Clamp block' (**Fig. 5.7**) of the connector cable is then fixed on to patient's thigh with the help of thigh belt (**Fig. 5.10**).

• Now remove the wax-seal from the ends of the two wires coming from the spiral electrode and clamp them in the two holes of the

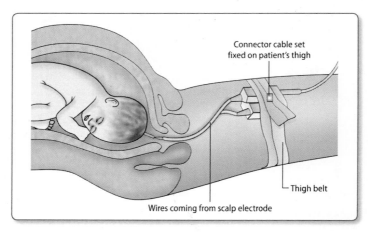

Fig. 5.10 Showing connections of scalp electrode

clamp block as shown in **Figure 5.10**. As this is done—the fetus gets connected with the machine.

- The power button on the machine is then switched on. As it is done, instantly, the machine shows the following functions— audible fetal heart sound, visible FHR display, and flashing of FHR lamp. In machines with the signal quality indicator light facility, the green 'OK' light also comes on signifying that the electrode is properly placed and anchored.
- Now, *switch the recorder* '**ON**' and note the quality of the tracing.

Technique of Operation of CTG Machine

- Internal CTG monitoring does not need any manual operation. It works automatically and uninterruptedly because the spiral electrode very rarely gets loose or comes off completely. This is in contrast to the external monitoring where the FH transducer often need resetting to cope with maternal and fetal movement.
- To economize on paper usage, the paper drive (the mechanism which produces the tracing on paper) may be operated intermittenly depending on the clinical gravity of the case.
- The volume of FHS may be adjusted as desired or may be put off completely.
- One has to be careful during vaginal examination so as not to dislocate the electrode from the presenting part. If dislocated, it has got to be reimplanted.

When to Remove the Electrode

1. It is the common practice to remove the scalp electrode with the crowning of the presenting part when the site of application is usually visible. However, in some units it is removed after complete delivery of the baby.
2. In case the patient is taken for cesarean section—removal has to be done just prior to the operation because, ideally, monitoring should continue until that time—specially in fetal distress cases. This can most conveniently be done with the help of Telemetry.

Alternatively, the CTG machine has to be wheeled to the OT and plugged in there.

Besides above the electrode may have to be removed at anytime during labor if application is improper as diagnosed by improper recording of FH. Under such circumstances it is removed and reapplied properly.

How to Remove the Electrode

Since the spiral type of electrode is fixed by clockwise rotation, it should be removed by anticlockwise rotation. It should never be pulled off by force because that will injure the scalp. No force is required for removal.

Fetal Arrhythmia and How to Record It

Some machines incorporate this special facility. Most CTG machines usually have an in-built logic which rejects beat-to-beat heart rate changes of more than 28 bpm. So, for recording the true rhythm of FH this logic facility must be made inoperative and then only arrthythmia if any, will show up. There, usually, is a special 'on/off switch for this facility which is operative—only with internal monitoring (i.e. with direct fetal ECG). **Fetal cardiac arrhythmia** has been reported in 3% of CTG tracings. Arrhythmia is defined as occurrence of episodes of bradycardia of less than 100 BPM, or tachycardia greater than 180 BPM between 30–40 weeks. However, most supraventricular arrhythmias are of little significance during labor unless there is coexistent heart failure as evidenced by Fetal hydrops (William's Obstetrics, 2010).

Some Operational Problems and their Solutions
Problems

The possible technical problems with internal monitoring are
- Intermittent FHR display
- Intermittent recording
- No display at all
- Continuous red light display on the signal quality indicator Window.

The Possible Causes

The cause of all these is either loose connection or no connection somewhere along the electrical line—from the scalp electrode—through the connector cable to the 'cardio' or 'ECG' socket on the CTG Machine.

Solution

The following are to be checked systematically:

a. Whether the cable plug is well inside the socket
b. Whether the electrode wires are well fixed to the clamp blocks of the connector cable
c. Whether the spiral electrode has become loose or has come off completely.

All these are easily correctable by the obstetric staff themselves. If all these are alright and still the FH recording is poor, the cause could be poor contact between the vaginal 'reference electrode' (**Fig. 5.6**) and the mother through the electrolytes present in her cervical and vaginal secretion. This problem can be solved by fixing an 'additional electrode' on the mother's upper thigh and connecting that to the clamp block of the connector cable set (**Fig. 5.10**) in place of the (red) wire coming from the original reference electrode already in place on the fetus.

Drawbacks of Internal Fetal Monitoring

1. It is invasive.
2. It needs much higher skill for its application.
3. It is more expensive than external monitoring. There is the recurring expense of buying electrodes.
4. It cannot be used on antenatal patients.
5. It cannot be used unless the cervix is adequately (2 cm) dilated
6. Chance of electrode dislocation during subsequent vaginal examinations necessitating reapplication.
7. Difficult to apply on fetus with thick hair.
8. May not be agreeable to some women – hurting the baby.

9. It immobilizes the patient unless telemery is used.
10. Small chance of fetal skin injury and bleeding.
11. Small chance of infection at the application site.
12. Very rare chance of maternal injury, if applied wrongly, on the cervix and then pulled off.

Special Advantages of Internal (CTG) Monitoring

1. Being ECG based it gives absolutely precise FHR.
2. By this method FHR recording is unaffected by the descent and rotation of fetus.
3. It is ideal for fetal monitoring in second stage of labor because it remains unaffected by the bearing down effort and other forms excessive movements on the part of the mother - in contrast to external method.

FURTHER READING

1. American College of Obst & Gyne (ACOG), Intrapartum Fetal Heart Monitoring, Practice Bulletin No. 70, December 2005. Quoted in William's Obstetrics, 23rd edition, 2010;410–43,
2. Carter MC, Gunn P, Beard RW. Brit J Obstet Gynaecol 1980;87:396–401.
3. Cunningham FG, Leveno KJ, Bloom SL, et al. In William's Obstetrics, 23rd Edition, Intrapartum Assessment, Mc Graw Hill, New York, 2010;410–43.
4. Dawes GS. Brit J Obstet Gynaecol, Vol.100, Supplement 1993;9:15–17.
5. Fraser DM and Cooper MA in Myles Textbook for Midwives, 15th Edition, Monitoring the Fetus, Churchill Livingstone, London, 2009;481–4.
6. Quinn A, Weir A, Shahani U, et al. Brit J Obstet Gynaecol 1994; 101:866–70.
7. Sonicaid TEAM Fetal monitor-user's guide: Publication No.8909-8500, Issue-2,1, Kimber Road, Oxford, UK, 1996;45–60.
8. Steer PJ. Fetal heart rate patterns and their clinical interpretation, Sussex, 1996; UK: Oxford Sonicaid Ltd. 1986;1–44.
9. Toitu CTG Machine brochure, foitu Co Ltd, 1-5-10,Ebisu-Nishi, Shibuya-Ku, Tokyo, Japan.

CHAPTER 6

Methods of Picking Up Uterine Activity—Tocography

Uterine activity, i.e. uterine contraction can be picked up by two methods–
1. External method
2. Internal method

EXTERNAL TOCOGRAPHY

Appliance Used

Pressure sensitive Tocodynamometer (transducer) of 'guard-ring'/strainguage type (**Fig. 6.1**).

Applicability

Can be used both for antenatal and intranatal monitoring of uterine contraction.

Mechanism of Working

The transducer senses the forward displacement of the uterus as the uterus contracts and depicts it in the form of tracing.

Practical Procedure of doing External Tocography

Fixing the Transducer

- Patient lies supine.
- The toco belt is arranged around her waist level so that the ends of the belt are on the top of the abdomen for fastening.

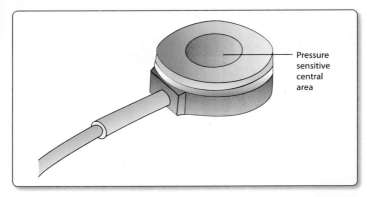

Pressure
sensitive
central
area

Fig. 6.1 Toco transducer or uterine contraction disc. This is used for external tocography

- Abdomen is then palpated to delineate the fundus of the uterus.
- The toco transducer plug is then plugged in the appropriate socket (Toco socket) on the CTG machine. The socket is usually, color matched, i.e. the socket and plug are of the same color. This is done in order to avoid confusion with 'cardio' plug and 'cardio' socket as described in previous chapters. On doing this, in some machine, TOCO-EXT sign lights up and the same words are annoted/printed on the chart paper.
- Toco transducer face—It is the side of the transducer that faces mother's abdomen. This surface with *central pressure sensitive area* is next placed on the fundus and fixed there with the help of the belt. It is best to choose a site where the distance between the transducer and the uterus is least. Difficult in obese patients.
- **No** gel or oil is required for its placement (**Fig. 6.1**).

Baseline Setting

Machines with external tocography facility have a uterine activity (UA) baseline setting button or a UA reference button. On pressing this and also the recorder (i.e. tracing drive) switch, the UA pen is set at a value of 10 in some Machines or 20 in some

Machines (see general description of CTG machine). It should be noted that this figure is not the value of intra-uterine basal tone. This is only a preset figure to fix a baseline so that the various features of contraction waves (e.g. its up-slope, peak, down-slope and baseline) are clearly depicted so as to be able to correlate them with the FHR pattern. Actually, it is so arranged in the machine that this figure is equivalent to the tension required to overcome the abdominal muscle artefact.

Reading the Trace on CTG Paper

As the uterus contracts the smaller bottom segment of the tracing paper depicts the wave of contraction—the various components of which have specific names as shown in **Figure 6.2**. (also read the chapter of "Uterine activity—normal and abnormal"—Chapter 16).

Information that can be Obtained by External Tocography

1. *The diagnosis whether the patient is contracting at all or not* This is of vital importance for making differentiation between false pain

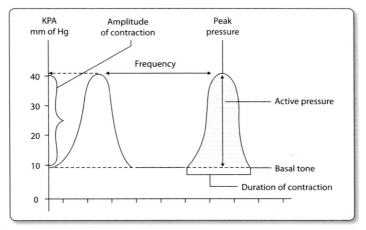

Fig. 6.2 Various component of a uterine contraction

and premature onset of labor because the management is entirely different. However, since "Uterine muscle efficiency to effect delivery varies greatly" one should be cautioned before judging the onset of true labor or its absence solely from the toco tracing (William's Obstetrics, 2010),.

It should be noted here that recording of frequent contraction on CTG does not always confirm that the patient is in labor because this can sometimes be seen in some patients who are not in clinical labor, i.e. who have no pain, whose os is closed or is not dilating progressively.

2. *The frequency of contraction*–This is a very useful information for management of labor. This tells the obstetrician in which case the labor is to be accelerated (e.g. a case of infrequent contraction). This also helps in adjustment of oxytocin drip rate.

3. *The duration of contraction*–This is a very important parameter of uterine contraction does not need overemphasis. This information is absolutely essential for interpreting FHR abnormalities in labor, e.g. early deceleration, late deceleration and variable deceleration. Besides, both short lived and prolonged contraction need attention (e.g. hyperstimulation).

External tocography offers only these three informations about uterine contraction and no more (see 'drawback' below). But, as can be easily judged, these are good enough for monitoring labor which is progressing satisfactorily (but, one may argue if a labor is progressing satisfactorily without any sign of fetal distress—what is the necessity of monitoring the contraction in such sophisticated way).

Actually, **the main reason** for monitoring contraction even when the labor is progressing satisfactorily—*is to see whether and how FHR is getting affected with the stress of uterine contraction.*

Hence, tocographic tracing **is a must** for giving real value to the method—the cardiotocography.

Drawbacks of External Tocography

1. It *cannot accurately measure* the following :
   a.   Amplitude of contraction.
   b.   Basal uterine tone.

   Due to the above deficiency external tocography is not good enough for monitoring slow labor or prolonged labor or where one wants to give relatively high dose of oxytocin. This is because these three clinical situations cannot be properly managed without the precise knowledge of the above two parameters of uterine contraction.

2. *Discomfort* of wearing toco belt constantly. Beltless transducer are being developed.

3. *Not very suitable for monitoring in second stage of labor as explained below.* External tocography produces rather too many *artifacts* specially in second stage of labor due to excessive movement of maternal abdominal muscles occasioned by maternal respiratory effort, her restlessness due to pain and to episodes of hyperventilation.

4. Produces artefact due to any movement of anterior abdominal wall, e.g. deep breathing, coughing, turning side in bed, etc.

INTERNAL TOCOGRAPHY

- Aim
- Scope
- Methods
- Drawbacks
- Place

Aim

Internal tocography aims to measure the intra-uterine pressure, i.e. changes in amniotic fluid pressure due to uterine contraction.

Scope

A postal survey conducted in UK showed that 70% of units did not have such a facility 20% did but used it infrequently and only 10%

used it frequently. It is estimated that overall less than 5% of all labors are candidates for internal tocometry (Gibb, 1993). More recently, this is what has been commented on internal Tocometry—"Direct intrauterine pressure monitoring is essentially only a research tool" (Magowan, 2009).

Methods Available

a. Fluid-filled intra-uterine catheter method—disposable.
b. Catheter-tip pressure transducer method—reusable (Sonicaid-Gaeltec).
c. Catheter cum pressure transducer method—disposable (Intran/Itran - Utah) with amnioport (see later)
   These three methods have been described in the next section.
d. Fiber optic device.

Fluid-Filled Intra-Uterine Catheter Method

- Materials required
- How to insert intra-uterine catheter
- Operation
- Technical problems and solution
- Disadvantage
   This technique used to be the most commonly used method but is being slowly replaced by the catheter-tip pressure transducer method (see later).

Materials required (See Figs 6.3 to 6.5)

1. Pressure transducer dome—disposable (**Fig. 6.3**).
2. Intra-uterine pressure kit—This consists of a long polythene intra-uterine catheter, a guide tube for catheter introduction, a 20 ml syringe, a special needle-adapter for connecting intra-uterine catheter and a three way stopcock. All these are disposable.
   Mounting hardware—This includes—screws, holder support, support pole, etc. (not disposable). The support pole is used for adjusting the level of the pressure transducer relative to that of maternal xiphoid (see later).

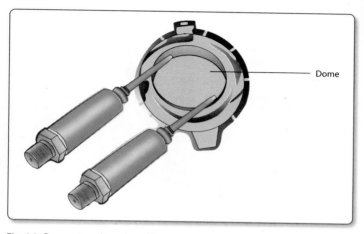

Fig. 6.3 Pressure transducer dome. This is connected at one end to the intra-amniotic pressure-catheter and at the other end to the CTG machine

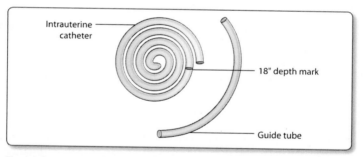

Fig. 6.4 Intrauterine catheter and guide tube (Introducer)

How to insert intrauterine catheter (Fig. 6.6)

- Do an aseptic vaginal examination.
- Pass up two fingers (middle and index) through the os between the posterior lip of cervix and the presenting part of the fetus for 4 or 5 cm.

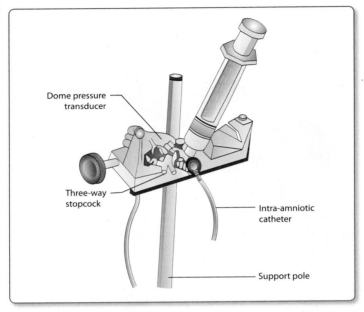

Fig. 6.5 Intra-uterine pressure kit for conventional intra-amniotic catheter. In this the pressure transducer remains outside (the mother's body) supported on a stand (support pole) so that its level can be adjusted relative to the level of xiphisternum of the mother. Changes in intra-uterine pressure is transmitted to the transducer through the fluid column in the intra-uterine catheter

- Now insert the 'guide tube' between the fingers following the curvature of pelvis and that of the presenting part for a short distance so that the tip of the guide tube lies just beyond the presenting part in the hind water when, automatically, the outer end of the tube would come to lie near your wrist. Because the tip of the guide tube lies in hind water, liquor starts draining through the guide tube as soon as it is inserted. Insertion of guide tube may be difficult with deeply engaged head.

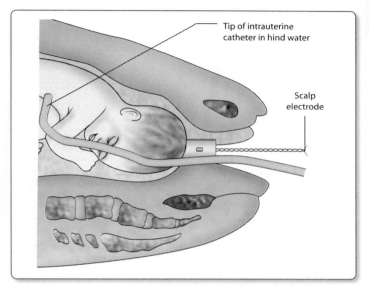

Fig. 6.6 Showing intrauterine catheter and scalp electrode *in situ*

- With the guide tube in place, insert the *perforated end* of the intra-amniotic catheter into the guide tube and gently advance it until '18 inch depth mark' on the catheter reaches the introitus.
- Now remove the guide tube by sliding it back on the catheter.
- Connect the end of the catheter with the 'special needle—adapter' provided and then connect this needle adapter to the 'three-way stopcock' provided and finally connect this stopcock to the 'pressure transducer dome' (**Fig. 6.7**). This dome is connected to the CTG machine through 'pressure transducer cable' by its plug.
- Fill a 20 ml syringe with distilled water and fit the syringe to the adapter of the three-way stopcock. Push 10 of distilled water into the intra-uterine catheter to make a continuous fluid column and also to free the catheter of all air. On pushing the piston-fluid should pass easily into the liquor amni.

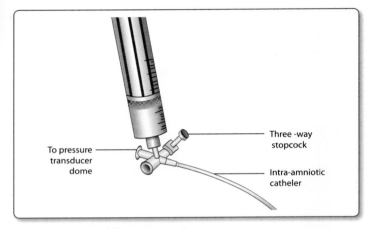

Fig. 6.7 Connections of three-way stopcock

- Close the stopcock to the syringe.
- Fix the whole thing on the 'holder support' provided (**Fig. 6.5**).
- Finally—Level the transducer with the maternal xiphoid. Some manufacturer recommend fixing of the transducer at the level of symphysis pubis.
- Once the pressure transducer has been plugged into CTG machine and the machine is switched on, ask the patient to cough and observe the spike on the contraction waveform to confirm optimal placement and function of the catheter.

Removal
The catheter may be removed when the second stage of labor commences because subsequent intra-uterine pressure level information is no longer accurate due to super addition of force of maternal bearing down effort.

Operation
The plug of the pressure transducer cable should be inserted into the TOCO socket of the CTG machine and then the recorder (trac-

ing drive) should be switched on for getting the tracing on paper. Zeroing should be done before taking reading. Zeroing cancels the atmosphere pressure to zero so as to eliminate it from the measured intra-uterine pressure.

Normally, the machine should show a basal tone of 8–12 mm of Hg.

Technical problems and solution

The common problems are:

i. *No pressure changes on toco numeric digital display during a contraction and non-appearance of wave form on tracing paper*—The possible causes of these may be:

    a. Obstruction in the catheter by vernix, etc. or

    b. Location of catheter tip in fluid-less environment or

    c. Dry catheter.

    The solution for all these would be to flush the catheter with sterile distilled water.

ii. *Pressure baseline is not visible –*

    This needs zero adjustment and also adjustment of the level of the transducer dome which should lie at the level of the xiphisternum.

Disadvantages of fluid-filled intrauterine catheter technique

1. Possibility of total blockage of the catheter with vernix, blood, etc. hence, no recording.

2. Danger of misinformation from partial blockage of catheter which then gives 'falsely low' reading which, in turn, may mislead the obstetrician to give excessive dose of oxytocin.

3. Baseline uterine tone reading is not always reliable because it depends upon the level of the pressure transducer dome relative to the upper fluid level in the uterus, which may vary with the mother's movement.

4. It is very cumbersome to set up and use the fluid-filled internal toco set because it consists of many small parts which must be fitted together. Then, there is the chance of some of these parts getting detached due to mother's movement.

5. It needs calibration before use.
6. It entails the recurring expenses of buying the intrauterine catheter set.
7. Any external factor which raises intra-abdominal and intrauterine pressure like coughing, heavy breathing, pushing, etc. cause artefact on the tracing. Sitting and using bedpan is a common example of external factor causing marked increase in intrauterine pressure.

Catheter tip pressure transducer method (Fig. 6.8) (Sonicaid-Gaeltec and others)

As the name implies here the pressure transducer is located at the tip of the intra-uterine catheter. This constitutes significant improvement over fluid filled intra-uterine catheter method offering the following relative advantages over it—

a. No complicated assembly is required. It is ever ready.
b. No calibration is required.
c. Being a solid catheter (!) no chance of blockage and consequent problems.
d. The problem about recording the basal tonus is avoided.
e. Since here the actual transducer lies within uterine cavity the readings are likely to be more accurate.

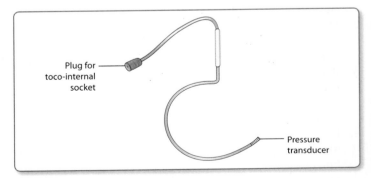

Plug for toco-internal socket

Pressure transducer

Fig. 6.8 Sonicaid-Gaeltec 'catheter-TIP' pressure transducer

However, the problem with this variety is—it is relatively fragile and hence unreliable for long-term use. Besides, it is more expensive.

Catheter cum Pressure Transducer Method with Amnioport (Fig. 6.9) (Intran)

Intran disposal intrauterine pressure catheter, though principly very similar to Gaeltec Catheter, differ from it in that it has a sheath-like introducer cum protector called 'protectaguide' and that it also provides an open communication channel into the amniotic sac called 'amnioport'. This latter facility allows:

a. Amnioinfusion to be delivered through it by attaching a drip set at its outer end and also

b. To perform amnioaspiration and wash in some cases of thickly meconium stained liquor.

The catheter is marked at 30 cm and 45 cm level. Normally, it should be introduced upto 45 cm level because, when this is done,

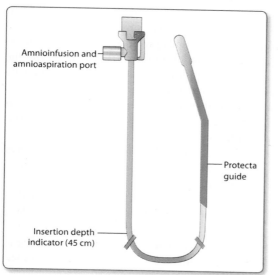

Amnioinfusion and amnioaspiration port

Protecta guide

Insertion depth indicator (45 cm)

Fig. 6.9 Intra-uterine catheter cum pressure transducer

i.e. when this mark comes to lie at introitus, the tip of the catheter lies at the fundus which is the correct place for it.

Drawbacks of Internal Tocometry

1. It is an invasive procedure.
2. It cannot be used for antenatal patients.
3. It requires membranes to be ruptured.
4. Small chance of perforation of the uterine wall by the guide tube.
5. Chance of injury to placenta, if it is posterior and somewhat low.
6. Risk of intra-uterine infection.
7. Requires a lot of skill.

Place of Internal Tocometry

1. For giving oxytocin stimulation in a post-cesarean case.
2. For giving oxytocin stimulation in a grand multipara.

   In both the instances the idea is to avoid rupture of the uterus through hyperstimulation.
3. For management of cases of unsatisfactory progress in the first stage of labor as defined by cervical dilation rate of less than 0.5 cm per hour inspite of contraction frequency of 5 per 10 min, occurring either spontaneously or with oxytocin stimulation (in absence of obstruction to the birth passage). Here the measurement of the ampitude of intrauterine pressure, specially the peak pressure, helps to diagnose precisely, whether it is a case of hypotonic inertia or otherwise and thereby help the obstetrician decide whether the case should be treated with higher concentration of oxytocin infusion or otherwise.

   An approach in this regard is to use oxytocin with external tocography until 12 mu/min. dosage thereafter if necessary to move on to internal tocography.

   Such objective approach helps both in reduction of cesarean rate and also that of unnecessary suffering of the mother in these cases.
4. In the cases where external tocometry is technically difficult, e.g. in grossly obese patients and restless patients. But for restless

patients the correct approach would be make the patient restful by appropriate medication and then to use external tocography.

5. For augmentation of labor in breech presentation—Though intrauterine pressure levels have been found to be similar in both spontaneous breech and spontaneous cephalic labor, some obstetrician prefer guidance of internal tocometry for augmentation of breech labor. However, nowadays most obstetricians prefer elective cesarean for breeches so no question of augmentation.

(Now read the chapter of—"Uterine activity—normal and abnormal"—Chapter 16).

UTERINE ELECTROMYOGRAPHY (EMG)

Currently, this is an experimental stage. This is an external method which has been designed to pick up the electrical activity of uterine muscle at the microscopic level.

It needs abdominal surface electrodes, electrical filters, amplifiers, signal acquisition hardware and analysis software (Nama and Arulkumaran, 2009).

Advantages of Uterine EMG

- It is a completely external method.
- Its measurements are comparable with those of intra-uterine pressure catheter while being *non-invasive*.
- May be able to predict the risk of preterm birth from as early as 27 weeks of pregnancy.

FURTHER READING

1. Gibb DMF. Brit J Obstet Gynaecol 1993;100(Supple)9:28–31.
2. Hewlett Packard Gmbh, D-7030, Boblingen: Operating Guide (1983) Technical information leaflets-1984 and 1986, Printed in the Federal Republic of Germany.
3. Magowan B, Owen P, Drife J: Clinical Obst Gynae, 2nd edition, Monitoring the Fetus in labor, Precipitate labor and Slow labor, Elsevier, Edinburg, 2009;331–43, 349–54.

4. Myles Textbook for Midwives:Edited by Fraser DM and Cooper MA, Monitoring the Fetus, Church Livingstone, London, 15th Edition, 2009;461–3, 472–3, 481–4, 487, 510–1, 518.

5. Nama V and Arulkumaran S: 'Uterine Contractions' in the book Best Practice in Labor and Delivery, Edited by Warren R and Arulkumaran S, 2009;54-65.

6. Sonicaid TEAM fetal monitor—User's guide: Publication No. 8909-8500, Issue-2,1, Kimber Road, Oxford, UK. 1996;54:63-9.

7. William's Obstetrics: 23rd Edition, Edited by Cunningham FG, Leveno KJ, Bloom SL, Hauth JC, Rouse DJ and Spong CY, Intrapartum Assessment, Mc Graw Hill, New York, 2010;437-43.

General Description of CTG Machine and its Various Switches, Control and Displays

Though the body of the machine, specially those which provide both internal and external monitoring facilities, may appear a bit complicated at first sight, on critical look specially from functional angle, it will turn out as a very simple machine. Here is a list of the various features of a standard CTG machine under broad headings.

1. Machine ON/OFF switch
2. Features concerned with fetal heart monitoring
3. Features concerned with uterine contraction monitoring
4. Switches for the recorder (paper drive)
5. Switches for annotation (for writing and marking)
6. LCD display facility
7. Memory
8. Home/Distance monitoring
9. Features of the CTG tracing paper
10. Arrangements for alram
11. Portability of CTG machine.

Please see **Figure 7.1** (the general CTG machine) in which some generalization has been made for easy understanding and for building a clear concept about any CTG machine of any make.

MACHINE ON/OFF SWITCH

This is actually power ON/OFF switch. Some machines' provide an indicator light which comes 'ON' when this switch is turned

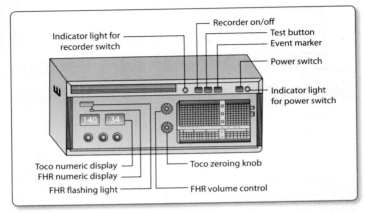

Fig. 7.1 General CTG machine

on. If the machine appears totally inoperative—examin this switch and also the main source of power—the simple fault (no power) may lie here.

FEATURES CONCERNED WITH FETAL HEART MONITORING

Features concerning FH monitoring depending on the make and model of the machine as follows:

a. *Sockect for ultrasonic FH transducer plug* – The socket and the plug usually have the same color to facilitate identification and avoid confusion so that the toco transducer (of different color) is not plugged in FH socket by mistake and vice versa. In some machines as the transducer is plugged in the socket an indicator light comes on to show that the plugging has been proper.

b. *Digital display of FHR* – This is a very prominent and important feature of the machine located on its front panel. By simply, glancing at this window one can judge from a distance the basic behaviour of FH e.g. tachycardia, bradycardia, etc.

c. *Flashing light display of FHR* – In addition to the digital display most machines also have a small light on the front panel which flashes in the rhythm of FH.

d. *FHR signal 'quality' display window* – Some machines incorporate this very useful facility in the design of traffic light signal—a window each for green, yellow and red light signifying optimal signal, fair signal and unacceptable signal respectively. This arrangement helps in:

   i. Proper positioning of the US transducer, i.e. right over FH—where external abdominal approach has been used for FH monitoring.

   ii. It also serves to indicate the right placement of scalp electrode, i.e. whether it is anchored properly—where the internal ECG mode has been used to pick up FH activity.

e. *FHS audio volume control knob* – This is useful in demonstrating FHS to the mother. A busy nurse in labour room can keep a tab on FH by raising its volume while doing other jobs.

f. *FHR abnormality 'alarm' bell/light* – Not all machines provide this. The alarm comes on when the normal range of FHR is exceeded. Obviously, for using this facility the desired upper and lower limits of FHR has to be preset (see later).

g. *Socket for 'direct' fetal ECG* – This is meant for the plug coming from the scalp electrode.

h. *FHR tracing on/off switch* – This is same as 'recorder switch' (see below) and is meant to drive (roll out) or stop the tracing paper. It also activates the pen which draws the tracing.

FEATURES CONCERNED WITH UTERINE CONTRACTION MONITORING

a. *Socket for TOCO Transducer* – Like the socket and plug for the ultrasonic FH transducer (see above) in this case also the socket and the transducer plug is color matched to avoid confusion with the FH transducer plug. Some machines have indicator light to show the mode that is being used to pick up uterine contraction (whether external or internal mode) which comes on as the socket is plugged in with the appropriate type of transducer. The TOCO socket is usually common for both internal (intra-amniotic catheter mode) and external (abdominal toco transducer mode) tocography.

b. *TOCO Baseline Setter Knob or Zeroing Knob* – This cancels the atmospheric pressure to zero so as to eliminate it from the measured intra-uterine pressure. For external tocography, it fixes the baseline to a preset level (see 'External tocography' in Chapter 6).

c. *TOCO Amplitude (i.e. Intra-Amniotic Pressure level) Numeric Display* – This shows the intra-unterine pressure level in Kpa or mm of Hg.

d. *TOCO Tracing on/off Switch* – This is same as 'recorder switch' (see below) and is common with FH tracing ON/OFF switch.

SWITCHES FOR THE RECORDER

The recorder is concerned with paper drive and pen drive so that the pens trace the events picked up by the machine on the paper in on-going manner. There are four switches concerned with the recorder as follows:

a. *Tracing on/off Switch* – On pressing this switch both FHR and toco pens start writing on the CTG tracing paper simultaneously and the paper also starts rolling out.

b. *Switch for the Manual Advancement of Paper* – This is required as one shifts the machine from one case to the next so as to be able to tear off the tracing of the last patient with a clear margin.

c. *Switch for Adjustment of Tracing Paper Speed* – Most machines give choice of three speeds: 1 cm, 2 cm and 3 cm per minute. This switch is usually located on one of the side panels or on the backside of the recorder assembly.

d. *Loading and Unloading of Tracing Paper* – It is quite simple but varies in details from one make of the machine to another. The manual book of each machine gives its own particular way.

PRINTER FACILITY

Some of the newer CTG machines have, a_ printer like the 'computer-printer'. The CT_ these machines is given out by this part of the sy_ conventional in-built recorder as in a conventiona_ Some of the sophisticated printers have even the *analys_* incorporated in it. So, these not only print the tracing _ result of the analysis of the issuing graph.

SWITCHES FOR ANNOTATION

These means switches for writing and marking on the CTG tracing paper, i.e. for making note.

a. *Automatic Annotation Facility* – Almost all machines with dual monitoring facility print the following data automatically— date, time, mode of picking up FH activity, (whether internal or external), mode of picking up uterine contraction (whether internal or external) and paper speed. This it does (usually) at 10 minutes interval on the narrow blank space at the junction of the FH portion and the TOCO portion of the tracing paper (see sample tracings in Chapter 13). These data are of great importance in analysing and following up of a case.

b. *Clinical Event Maker Button* – On pressing this button an arrow or some other sign (varies with the machine) gets printed on the tracing paper to mark some clinical event like the point of time when acoustic stimulation was given, membranes were ruptured, meconium first appeared, etc. This button is, usually located right on the body of the machine.

c. *Remote Event Maker* – This is a switch at the end of a long flex which is plugged into the appropriate socket on the CTG machine. This switch is given to the mother when she is having her CTG done. She is instructed to press the switch as and when she feels fetal movement and as soon as she presses the switch, depending on the make of the machine either an arrow or a thin

ther sign get printed on
t that point. It is from
and the occurrence of
switch is also called by

which have a socket for
sign of musical note on
ulator switch is pressed

part of it, a detachable
tracing on paper in
m instead of the
TG machine.
ic software
also the

e front panel which displays all monitoring parameters on real time including the graphs. This has the major advantage of doing continuous monitoring but without paper, i.e. it saves expensive paper. If obstetrician desires to permanently record any segment of the tracing on display it can be done by simply pressing the recorder switch. Undoubtedly, this is a very useful facility

MEMORY

Some newer machines have storage capacity (memory) of holding six hours data—both alphanumeric and graphic. So, CTG monitoring done on a patient some hours or days back but without paper tracing can be called back and, if necessary, be printed, at any time. Through this facility data of many patients can be stored in one machine.

This facility is of particular advantage for home monitoring. CTG of several patients can be taken by a junior doctor or an obstetric nurse at patients home and then when the machine is brought back to hospital the tracings taken earlier at home can be accessed for analysis by a senior doctor who can also match the CTG findings with patients clinical data which is available at the hospital.

HOME/DISTANCE MONITORING

See chapter 28 on Telemetry.

FEATURES OF CTG TRACING PAPER

A clear knowledge about the format of the CTG tracing paper is important for prompt and correct interpretation of the tracings that come on it. But, unfortunately, this most simple and basic component of CTG procedure has not yet been standardized—each manufacturer using a slightly different format. Here is a summary of the basic features of CTG tracing paper.

Paper Width

For most makes of the machine, the paper width is more of less around 150 mm but the chart papers are not interchangeable between one make of the machine to another.

Recording Channels

Basically, all machines have 2 channels as follows:

- Top channel (80 mm)—This is for FHR recording.
- Bottom channel (40 mm)—This is for uterine contraction recording/(Toco channel)

Machines with dual FHR monitoring facility for twins depicts and prints the FHR traces of two fetuses a) either one above the other in which case the FHR channel is divided into an upper and lower half of 40 mm each with one half for each fetus b) or prints them together across the full 80 mm width of the FHR channel like this – of that of one fetus *in dark* and that of the other *in light ink.*

About the facility for automatic printing (every ten minutes) of date, time, monitoring mode and paper speed—the details have already been mentioned above. These are printed in the blank space between the FHR and the toco channel.

Machines with actocardiograph facility print occurrence of fetal movement either in 'dot print' or as 'tiny black squares' near the upper border of either FHR channel or Toco channel or 'as grassy marks (spikes)' near the bottom of the Toco channel (see **Fig. 13.49**).

FHR range—As Printed on the Chart Paper
Papers of some monitors print—50–210 bpm
Papers of some monitors print—30–240 bpm

Steps of FHR Increment and Decrement Depiction
(as denoted by the distance between the horizontal lines on the chart paper).
See **Figure 7.2** and the actual tracings in the Chapter 13.

This is a very important feature and can cause a lot of confusion in interpretation of the tracings because interpretation is generally done by 'visual impression' of the size of the humps and depressions of the FHR tracing line. The confusion occurs under the following situations.

i.   When one unit has two machines of two different companies using papers of two different specifications.

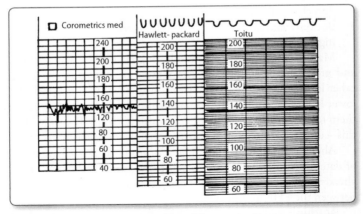

Fig. 7.2 Showing a slice of FHR chart of three different makes. Note how different they are

ii. When the same patient is monitored by a machine of one make one day and another make another day—each using their own brand of tracing paper.

iii. When an obstetrician, who is used to chart paper of one make of CTG machine, happens to judge or compare the tracing coming out of machine of another make using another kind of paper.

Given below is a comparison of chart paper (FHR channel only) of three different manufacturers (also see **Fig. 7.2**).

Table 7.1

Names of Company	Steps of FHR as printed on chart	No. of horizontal lines in between two printed FHR figures	BPM interval between two consecutive horizontal lines
Hewlett Packard (HP)	Step of 20 bpm e.g. 100, 120, 140 etc.	4 lines	5 bpm
Corometrics	Step of 30 bpm e.g. 90, 120, 150 etc.	3 lines	10 bpm
Toitu	Step of 20 bpm e.g. 100, 120, 140 etc.	10 lines	2 bpm

See Figure 7.2 showing a slice each of the three types of charts. Note: Features vary from model to model of the same company.

It is quite apparent from the above table how confusing it is to compare three charts of three different machines, specially visually, and hence, there is an urgent need for standardization of the chart paper internationally.

Paper Features of TOCO Tracing

Here also there is some non-uniformity as shown in **Figure 7.3**. Whereas, the amplitude of contraction is depicted in either mm of

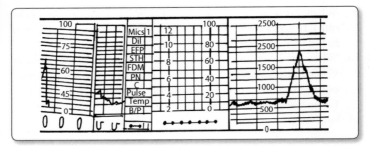

Fig. 7.3 Showing a slice of toco chart of four kinds. They seems to be so different

Hg or KPA or in both in papers of some make some others do not print the unit of measurement at all.

Though unrelated to actual tocography, some manufactures use the toco section of the paper to provide columns for entering the observations like—dilatation of cervix, effacement, station, state of membranes, mother's pulse, temperature, BP, medication given, PH of fetal blood, oxymetry findings, etc. for labour cases.

Paper Speed

Unfortunately, between manufactures, there is no uniformity in this feature either. While some companies give a choice of three speeds, i.e. 1 cm/min, 2 cm/min. and 3 cm/min., some other companies offer only two choices—1 cm and 3 cm/min. One can well imagine how different 'the same FHR tracing would look if run first on 1 cm/min and then on 3 cm/min speed and the consequent diagnostic problem.

Recommendation

Working party on 'cardiotocography technology' organized by the Royal College of Obstetricians and Gynecologists of London recommend the following for FHR display in CTG : A range of 50 to 210 bpm at 20 bpm/cm scale sensitivity and a paper speed of 1 cm/min., so that the visual appearance of the recording would be the same irrespective of the make of the machine used (Carter and Steer, 1993).

ARRANGEMENT FOR ALARM

For FHR

a. In some machines one can set *rate base alarm* for a chosen lower and higher limit of FHR, e.g. at 110 bpm and at 160 bpm.

b. In some machines there is arrangement for *signal loss base alarm* so that if there occurs FH signal loss exceeding 30% in any 10 min period, alarm goes so that one attends the case to set the problem right. Two common causes of signal loss are—change in fetal position and hence, that of its heart and transducer or scalp electrode displacement.

For Toco

Some machines have arrangement so that alarm goes *if no contraction is recorded for a continuous period of 10 minutes* so that, due attention may be given to the case.

The possible causes of non-recording of contractions and their solutions are –

a. Toco disc displacement—needs repositioning,

b. Intrauterine pressure catheter displacement—needs repositioning,

c. Truely infrequent contraction (= Slow labor) i.e. stimulation of contraction by oxytocic may be considered.

d. A possible case of 'false pain' consider necessary treatment.

e. A possible case of premature labor institute appropriate treatment.

Portably of CTG Machine

All CTG machines are portable on their own trolley or any other trolley. But in the recent years most manufacturers have reduced the dimensions and weight of the machine to such an extent that they can be easily carried in hand. Size has been reduced to roughly 10–12" in all dimensions—width height and depth, and the weight also reduced to less than 2 kg. Some manufacturers have even separated the printer which now may or may not be carried to the patient. In these models one can see the tracing on LCD screen, store the whole recording in the memory and later have it printed if required.

Advantages of Portability

The very small machines which can be carried in hand has the following advantages–

1. By one machine one can cover many locations like antenatal clinic, antenatal ward and labor room.

2. For patients who should not be moved like—APH patients, hypertension patients under heavy sedation, cases of threatened premature labor, etc. the machine can be taken to patients bedside. Similarly, for emergency cases, it can be taken to emergency room.

3. For IUGR patients who cannot afford admission to hospital or nursing home and who must rest—the machine can be carried to patient's home. In fact, this way hospital admission and thereby overcrowding of hospital can be reduced.

4. As the machine hardly takes any space—it is ideal for private chamber (office) of the obstetrician where the space available is usually limited.

    Note: Carrying the machine in hand is usually better than wheeling it on a trolley with illfitted wheels and specially where stairs have to be negotiated.

FURTHER READING

1. Analogic FetalGard Lite CTG machine-NIBP, Analogic Corporation, USA, 2003.

2. BPL Fetal Monitor- 9533, Fetal cum Maternal Monitor-FM 9714, BPL Healthcare, Bangalore, India.

3. Carter MC, Steer PJ. Brit J Obstet Gynaecol 1993;100(Supple)9:1–36.

4. Corometrics Fetal monitor—Model 145 Operator's manual: Corometrics Medical systems, INC; 61 Barnes Park Road, North Walingford , Connecticut, USA-06492, 1992;1–27. Now represented by GE USA, 2005

5. Hewlett Packard Gmbh D-7030, Boblingen: Operating guide for fetal monitor Model 8040A and Technical information leaflets 1984 and 1986 Printed in the Federal Republic of Germany, 1983;84:86., Now represented by Philips, Netherland, 2002.

6. Huntleigh Fetal Monitors, Baby Dopplex 4000, Cardiff, UK, 2007.

7. Philips Fetal Monitors, Netherland : Antepartum Monitor-FM-2, M-1351A, Intrapartum Fetal Monitor- Series 50 IP-2, 2010.

8. Sonicaid-Fetal heart rate patterns and their clinical interpretations Oxford Sonicaid Ltd, Quarry Lane, Chichester, W Sussex, UK, 1986;1–45.

9. Sonicaid Team Fetal Monitor-user's Guide: Publication No 8909-8500, UK, P-45-73, 99–111, 143–144,1996, 2006

10. Toitu CTG Machine brochure and Toitu guide to fetal heart rate monitoring, ToituCo Ltd, 1-5-10, Ebisu-Nishi, Shibuya-Ku, Tokyo, 150 Japan.

How to Choose a Machine

Given below a 'facility cum suitability-based classification' of CTG machine so as to help a prospective buyer to choose the right machine for his/her requirement and budget.

a. Machines meant for 'external'monitoring only.
b. Machines meant for 'both' external and internal monitoring.
c. Machines with special 'twin monitoring' facility.
d. Machines with automatic fetal movement profile monitoring facility (Actocardiography).
e. Machines with facility for automatic 'computer analysis and interpretation' of the tracing.
f. Machines with 'telemetry' facility.
g. Combined fetal and maternal monitoring system.
h. CTG machine with water-resistant transducers – for under water delivery.
i. CTG machine without in-built recorder/printer.

MACHINES MEANT FOR 'EXTERNAL' MONITORING ONLY

In these machines FH activity is picked up by US Doppler mechanism from the mother's abdomen. These have no fetal electrocardiography facility—direct or indirect. Toco pick-up element is also applied externally on the abdomen.

These machines are usually quite small and portable, and is ideal for NST, CST, VAST, etc. These are well-suited for obstetrician's private chamber and antenatal clinics. The great advantage of this variety is—it can be used for both *antenatal* and *intranatal* monitoring. These are least expensive.

MACHINES MEANT FOR BOTH 'EXTERNAL AND INTERNAL' MONITORING

These machines provide 'double mode of recording' facility for both FH and uterine activity.

For Picking-up FH Activity

These provide, (a) US Doppler transducer for external (abdominal) monitoring and (b) direct fetal ECG facility through fetal scalp electrode for internal (through vagina) monitoring.

For Picking-up Uterine Activity

These provide (a) abdominal US pressure transducer for external (abdominal) monitoring and (b) intrauterine catheter for internal (vaginal) pick-up of intra-amniotic pressure changes.

These machines are best-placed in the labor room for its full utilization because the internal monitoring facility can be used only in labour and only after the membranes have ruptured or have been ruptured. It is ideal for institutions, specially those units who deal with lots of complicated and high risk cases who are best-monitored internally by placement of scalp electrode.

These equipments are more expensive (roughly double in price) in comparison to "external only" machines.

MACHINES WITH SPECIAL 'TWIN MONITORING' FACILITY

Hardware-wise, these machines are very similar to the last variety of machines with dual (both internal and external) monitoring facility.

The only extra-component present in these is—they have arrangements within the machine for 'simultaneous' dual heart monitoring and recording facility which entails providing two separate FH monitoring sockets instead of one—one meant for Doppler US transducer and the another for direct fetal ECG. The idea is, during labour, after the rupture of membranes, the presenting twin can be monitored through the placement of fetal electrode and the other, abdominally, by the US transducer.

Newer CTG machines now have the facility for *'non-invasive, totally external, antenatal monitoring of twin'* pregnancy. Oxford Sonicaid TEAM - S8000 printer also provides dual channel (for twins) printing *with simultaneous analysis* but it needs two Team-base units for the purpose.

As regards the price one has to pay extra for the extra-facility.

(Also see Chapter 27—'Monitoring twins by CTG' later).

MACHINES WITH AUTOMATIC FETAL MOVEMENT PROFILE MONITORING FACILITY

These machines use abdominal US transducer to monitor FM which automatically gets traced on the chart in toco channel portion of the chart. Naturally, these machines give extremely good NST, i.e. precise picture of **FM acceleration** (Also read the special section—'Fetal actocardiogram/Actogram' later in Chapter 15).

MACHINES WITH AUTOMATIC 'COMPUTER ANALYSIS AND INTERPRETATION' FACILITY

See the exclusive chapter on it—Chapter 20.

MACHINES WITH TELEMETRY FACILITY

See the exclusive chapter on it—Chapter 28. Obviously, this is a model for very busy obstetric units having many machines working simultaneously.

CTG MACHINE WITH WATER RESISTANT TRANSDUCERS

Marmaid model of CTG machine (Spacelab Medicals) have transducers which are water resistant. So, the patient can have bath in bath tub or shower while still getting monitored. This is ideal for women who desire under water delivery and where such facility is available.

CTG MACHINE WITHOUT RECORDER

Some latest models of CTG machines have done away with the standard in-built recorder system which needs tailor-made proprietary tracing paper—an item which is expensive and not always easy to get. Instead, they have so modified the technology by adding a new software that the tracing can now be taken on any ordinary 'computer printer ' which is quite a cheap item and uses normal readily available ordinary cheap printing paper. One can, in fact, now use ones own already existing computer printer. If one chooses such a model, the price of CTG machine and its running cost come down significantly.

RECOMMENDATION FOR STORAGE OF TRACINGS

These are best stored in 'Soft' form in CDs or Pen drive in PDF form. This storing method has the following advantages – a) needs very little storage space, b) easily transferable anywhere electronically. Besides, tracings taken on the thermal paper tend to fade away and of course these are voluminus.

Combined Fetal and Maternal Monitoring System

This is the new trend which aims at perfection.

These machines, in addition to giving both external and internal mode of CTG, also simultaneously and automatically record and depict on the screen, and if required on paper, *all the vital basic parameters of mother as well,* e.g. her pulse, temperature, respiration, her ambulatory blood pressure (NIBP), SpO_2 and ECG if needed.

These versatile machines are ideal for big institutions and referral centers and are extremely useful in managing patients with medical disorders like heart disease, asthma, severe anemia, eclampsia etc.

These not only a) improve the quality of monitoring but also b) save time and c) manpower requirement.

FURTHER READING

1. Analogic FetalGard Lite CTG machine-NIBP, Analogic Corporation, USA, 2003.

2. BPL Fetal Monitor- 9533, Fetal cum Maternal Monitor-FM 9714, BPL Healthcare, Bangalore, India.

3. Carter MC, Steer PJ. Brit J Obstet Gynaecol 1993;100(Supple)9:1–36.

4. Corometrics Fetal monitor—Model 145 Operator's manual: Corometrics Medical systems, INC; 61 Barnes Park Road, North Walingford , Connecticut, USA-06492, 1992;1–27. Now represented by GE USA, 2005

5. Hewlett Packard Gmbh D-7030, Boblingen: Operating guide for fetal monitor Model 8040A and Technical information leaflets 1984 and 1986 Printed in the Federal Republic of Germany, 1983;84:86., Now represented by Philips, Netherland, 2002.

6. Huntleigh Fetal Monitors, Baby Dopplex 4000, Cardiff, UK, 2007.

7. Philips Fetal Monitors, Netherland : Antepartum Monitor-FM-2, M-1351A, Intrapartum Fetal Monitor- Series 50 IP-2, 2010.

8. Sonicaid-Fetal heart rate patterns and their clinical interpretations Oxford Sonicaid Ltd, Quarry Lane, Chichester, W Sussex, UK, 1986;1–45.

9. Sonicaid Team Fetal Monitor-user's Guide: Publication No 8909-8500, UK, P-45-73, 99–111, 143–144,1996, 2006

10. Toitu CTG Machine brochure and Toitu guide to fetal heart rate monitoring, ToituCo Ltd, 1-5-10, Ebisu-Nishi, Shibuya-Ku, Tokyo, 150 Japan.

Electrical Requirement and Environment

POWER SOURCES AND CONSUMPTION

CTG machines need AC current sources with voltage of 115 or 230 volts. Some machines have voltage selector switch so that one can select right voltage appropriate to one's supply. Voltage stabilizer is required only in areas where supply voltage is known to fluctuate widely.

Power Consumption

It is very low—around 50 watts.

Earthing Facility

Always use three pin plug with good earthing facility.

PRECAUTIONS

- Make sure that the patient's cable must not come into contact with any other electrical equipment or with the metal bed-frame.
- To avoid leakage of current—transducer gel, electrode gel or any other wet substance should not be kept on the monitor.
- The machine should not be used in presence of inflammable anesthetics.

ROOM TEMPERATURE

The CTG machine need not be kept in airconditioned room. It can work at the ambient temperature between 10° to 35°C.

ELECTROMAGNETIC INTERFERENCE

It is necessary to ensure that the area in which the CTG machine is kept is not subject to any sources of strong electromagnetic interference such as radio-transmitters, mobile phones, etc.

FURTHER READING

1. Analogic FetalGard Lite CTG machine-NIBP, Analogic Corporation, USA, 2003.
2. BPL Fetal Monitor- 9533, Fetal cum Maternal Monitor-FM 9714, BPL Healthcare, Bangalore, India.
3. Carter MC, Steer PJ. Brit J Obstet Gynaecol 1993;100(Supple)9:1–36.
4. Corometrics Fetal monitor—Model 145 Operator's manual: Corometrics Medical systems, INC; 61 Barnes Park Road, North Walingford, Connecticut, USA-06492, 1992;1–27. Now represented by GE USA, 2005
5. Hewlett Packard Gmbh D-7030, Boblingen: Operating guide for fetal monitor Model 8040A and Technical information leaflets 1984 and 1986 Printed in the Federal Republic of Germany, 1983;84:86., Now represented by Philips, Netherland, 2002.
6. Huntleigh Fetal Monitors, Baby Dopplex 4000, Cardiff, UK, 2007.
7. Philips Fetal Monitors, Netherland : Antepartum Monitor-FM-2, M-1351A, Intrapartum Fetal Monitor- Series 50 IP-2, 2010.
8. Sonicaid-Fetal heart rate patterns and their clinical interpretations Oxford Sonicaid Ltd, Quarry Lane, Chichester, W Sussex, UK, 1986;1–45.
9. Sonicaid Team Fetal Monitor-user's Guide: Publication No 8909-8500, UK, P-45-73, 99–111, 143–144,1996, 2006
10. Toitu CTG Machine brochure and Toitu guide to fetal heart rate monitoring, ToituCo Ltd, 1-5-10, Ebisu-Nishi, Shibuya-Ku, Tokyo, 150 Japan.

CHAPTER 10

Machine Testing by the User

This means day-to-day testing of the machine as a matter of routine when it is in use or about to be used after a rest period and also in the event of its malfunctioning.

COMPREHENSIVE SELF-TESTING

For this, some machines have a button called 'test button' which on pressing self-tests all the important functions of the machine like—displays, recorders, speakers, etc. and also all its internal circuitory and calibration. However, most newer machines, automatically does this comprehensive self-testing every time the machine is switched on.

TESTING ULTRASONIC FH TRANSDUCER

Actually every time the 'test button test' is performed as above, the transducer gets indirectly tested by the process of exclusion, i.e. if comprehensive self-testing shows everything inside the machine is alright and still the machine is not functioning properly—one can assume that the defect perhaps lies in the transducer rather than the body of the machine.

Most manufacturers give their own method of testing the Ultrasonic FH Transducer. However, three simple techniques of doing this are described below.

Technique I

After plugging in the transducer cable and keeping the volume control in middle position, the transducer disc has to be held in front of the palm of the other hand. Then this other hand is to be repeatedly moved toward and then away from the transducer face (**Fig. 10.1**). On doing so, if a synchronised noise is heard from the loud speaker it signifies that the transducer is alright.

Technique II

A little bit of aquasonic gel is to be applied on the palm of left hand (the test may be done even without the gel) and the transducer has to be held in this hand with its face in contact with the gel on the palm. Then, after switching on the machine, the back of the hand holding the transducer is to be rubbed repeatedly with the index finger of the right hand in high speed (**Fig. 10.2**). While doing this—one should listen to the audio-output (the sound), look at the pulse lamp, the FHR digital display and the tracing paper. It will be found that all

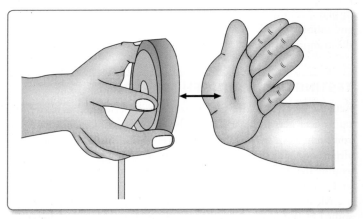

Fig. 10.1 Testing US fetal heart transducer by moving the palm toward and then away from the transducer face

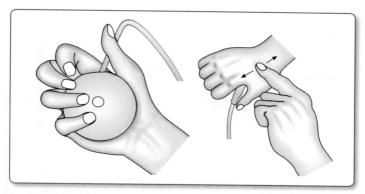

Fig. 10.2 Testing US fetal heart transducer by repeatedly rubbing the back of the hand holding the transducer

these parameters are giving synchronised signals proportionate to the speed of the finger movement. If this happens the transducer and the whole system can be certified to be functioning normally.

Technique III

This is a very useful test to know whether the piezo-crystals (seven numbers) housed in the US transducer (**Fig. 10.3**) got dislocated or not which can occur if it happens to fall from hand or gets any hard knock. Since the crystals are not externally-visible they have to be tested blindly by approximation one-by-one. For this, after plugging in the transducer and switching on the machine, a blob of aquasonic gel has to be put on the face of the transducer disc at any point near its periphery (**Fig. 10.3**) and then, keeping the gel tube in contact with the transducer through the gel blob, the tube has to be moved up and down rapidly over the approximate site of each crystal one-by-one. Variation in sound in synchronism with the tube movement indicates that the crystals have not been displaced and the transducer is alright.

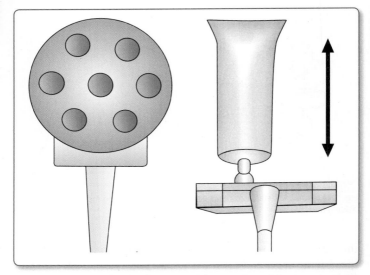

Fig. 10.3 Showing a technique of testing any dislocation of any of the piezo- electric crystals in a US fetal heart transducer which can happen if the transducer accidently falls from hand or gets a hard knock

TESTING TOCO TRANSDUCER

This can be easily performed by gently pressing its central pressure-sensitive part. As it is being done an eye should be kept on both the uterine activity (UA) channel of the tracing paper and also on the UA numerical display window on the machine. If the toco transducer is functioning alright both these displays will register increase of pressure.

Actually, transducers need to be individually-tested only if there is any malfunction inspite of normal reading on 'test button test' or auto-testing as described above.

BIBLIOGRAPHY

1. Hewlett Pacard Gmbh, Boblingen. Operating guide for fetal monitor. Model 8040A and Technical information leaflets-1984 and 1986, printed in the Federal Republic of Germany. 1983;84:86.
2. Sonicaid TEAM fetal Monitor user's guide: Publication No 8909-8500, Issue 2,1, Kimber road, Oxford, UK. 1996;45–73, 99–111, 143–4.

Machine Servicing

SELF-SERVICING

This has two components namely:
1. Basic care in the use of machine, and
2. Regular cleaning

Basic Care

a. Transducer must be handled gently and carefully because a fall or a bang may damage the delicate piezo-electric crystals inside.

b. The cable attached to the transducer should not be flexed excessively since it may cause damage to the wire inside.

c. Avoid using alcohol-based, ammonia-based or acetone-based cleaners; also avoid using strong antiseptics like Lysol, concentrated povidone iodine, etc. because these may corode or stain the monitor.

d. Do not ever immerse transducer and connector in water.

e. To protect from dust and accidental damage it is best to make a cabinet for the machine keeping 15 cm space all round for dissipation of heat.

Regular Cleaning

Wipe all 'external surfaces' with mild detergent dissolved in distilled water (never use saline because this is an electrolyte solution). Avoid using very hot water. After cleaning, wipe with dry cloth to make everything dry. Once a week cleaning is usually enough.

Re-usable belts should be washed with soap and water and then with diluted Savlon for disinfection.

All components of the monitor which must go inside the body of the patient like scalp electrode, intra-uterine catheter set, etc. should better be of disposable type.

Internal cleaning must be done only by professional service engineers.

Sterilization

Sterilization of this equipment is not normally required. However, if ever required the only method to be used both for the case and the transducers is ethylene oxide gas upto 5.5 bar (see also manufcturer's guide)

PROFESSIONAL-SERVICING

This should be done at four months interval (three times a year) and it is best to have service contract with the dealer for this purpose.

CTG Interpretation—Theoretical Considerations

(This chapter contains *the mind or the brain* of the whole CTG procedure and should be studied very carefully. One will have to often refer back to this chapter while studying the tracings given in the next chapter and also, may be, for interpretation of the tracings from an actual case in practice).

FEATURES TO SEE IN A CTG TRACING

The following seven features are to be critically observed in any CTG tracing:

1. Baseline FHR
2. Baseline variability of FHR
3. Any acceleration of FHR
4. Any deceleration
5. Incidents associated with acceleration or deceleration if any like—with fetal movement, uterine contraction, etc.
6. Uterine contraction, where present—their frequency, duration and amplitude and also the basal uterine tone, i.e. the tone in between contractions. The last two parameters can only be assessed where internal tocometry through placement of intrauterine catheter has been used.
7. Precise *time-correlation* of FH changes with the onset, peak and disappearance of uterine contraction.

In addition to above, special analysis is required for cases where stimulation tests have been done like • Acoustic stimulation, • Scalp stimulation, etc.

This chapter has been presented in six separate sections as follows in order to deal with these very important parameters in reasonable detail:

a. Baseline FHR—General considerations
b. Tachycardia
c. Bradycardia
d. Baseline variability of FHR
e. Accelerations
f. Decelerations

BASELINE FHR—GENERAL CONSIDERATIONS
CTG Definition of Baseline FHR

Baseline FHR on a CTG tracing is taken as the mean FHR over a period and should be arrived at by observing a tracing of at least *10 minutes duration*. It is deduced from continuous FHR record by imagining a line passing horizontally, roughly, *through the 'middle'* of the wavy line of the FH tracing (**Fig. 12.1**) indicating sort of average rate of FH between the upper and lower limits of it's variability.

Clinical definition

Clinically baseline FHR is taken as the rate found on ordinary auscultation at any given point of time, and time to time.

Note

Baseline FHR is difficult to record in cases of arrhythmia. About 'doubling' and 'halving' error of baseline FHR—details have already been given in Chapter 5. Such error is possible only with external (ultrasonic) method of FHR monitoring and not with internal (ECG) method of monitoring.

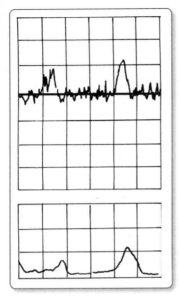

Fig. 12.1 A horizontal line has been drawn through the middle of the wavy line of FH tracing indicating sort of average rate of FH, i.e. the baseline rate. Notice two typical healthy accelerations of more than 15 BPM and lasting more than 15 seconds. Also notice that these two accelerations have coincided with uterine contraction (see text)

Normal Baseline FHR at Various Periods of Gestation

12–30 Weeks –	140–180 BPM
30–40 Weeks –	120–160 BPM
40+ Weeks –	Lowest upto 110 BPM may be considered as normal (see below)

This reduction in FHR with increasing maturity is brought about by the increasing maturity of the fetal vagal center.

Norms of Baseline FHR for CTG

- Classical view
  - Normal range –   120–160 BPM
  - Tachycardia –   More than 160 BPM
  - Bradycardia –   Less than 120 BPM
- FIGO view (1987)
  - Normal range –   110–150 BPM

Other View (Arulkumaran, 1992)

Rate between 100–110 (moderate bradycardia) and between 150–170 (moderate tachycardia) can be taken as normal—provided the trace shows accelerations, normal baseline variability and no deceleration (and provided the liquor is not meconium stained).

Neurohormonal Control of Baseline FHR
Autonomic Nervous Control
Parasympathetic

Parasympathetic nerves have been demonstrated in FH at, as early as, eighth week of gestation. As expected, stimulation of parasympathetic nervous system causes bradycardia. As already mentioned parasympathetic vagal centre matures with increasing fetal maturity.

Sympathetic

Naturally, stimulation of sympathetic causes tachycardia.

The two systems remains in fine balance with one taking the upper hand for a few moments and the other taking upper hand for the next few moments and hence the heart rate varies constantly in a fetus and produces an irregular saw-toothed appearance on CTG trace (see 'short-term variability' and (**Fig. 12.2**).

It is noteworthy that there exists some difference in the tempo of action between the two systems—whereas parasympathetic stimulation causes instant bradycardia (see Type 1 dip), with sympathetic stimulation the rate of rise of FHR is rather slow.

Receptor mechanism

Just to briefly recapitulate—changes in FHR is mediated via two kinds of receptors located in aortic and carotid sinus.

  a. *Baroreceptors:* These contain stretch receptors and are designed to respond to fetal blood pressure changes (as in cord compression):
  • Rise of BP: This induces bradycardia by stimulating parasympathetic (vagal) activity.
  • Fall of BP: This causes tachycardia by inhibiting vagal activity.

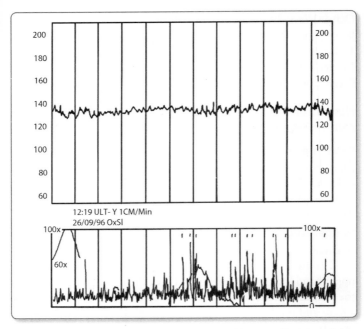

Fig. 12.2 Notice the irregular saw-toothed appearance of FH tracing. This is brought by the fine interplay between sympathetic and parasympathetic on FH. Also note that the baseline variability is very poor here (only 2-3 BPM)

b. *Chemoreceptor:* These mainly respond to PO_2 of blood. In addition to carotid sinus (the peripheral receptor site) some of these chemoreceptors are also present in brainstem (the central receptor site). While the peripheral receptors are activated by hypoxemia the central ones are affected by (more severe) 'tissue hypoxia' of brain.

Humoral Control

Really, only two hormones influence FHR—they are Adrenalin and Noradrenalin. Both maternal and fetal stress cause tachycardia through this mechanism.

Types of Baseline Abnormality

Baseline abnormalities are of three types:

- Tachycardia
- Bradycardia
- Baseline variability

TACHYCARDIA

Baseline tachycardia means sustained (not transient) increase in FHR to above 160 bpm. Such label should be put on only after observing the tracing for a minimum period of *10 minutes*.

Causes of Baseline Tachycardia
Stress

Adrenaline and noradrenalin released by mother or fetus in response to stressful stimuli have a powerful effect on FHR causing tachycardia.

However, if the stress is severe causing release of a very high quantity of catecholamine, it may cause constriction of uterine blood vessels, interfering with the placental blood supply leading to hypoxic bradycardia (Steer, 1986).

Mother in severe pain with resultant increase in her sympathetic tone may also excite fetal tachycardia which usually settles on giving adequate analgesia (Ingemarsson, et al. 1993).

Hypoxia

In a case of gradually developing hypoxia, the baseline FHR gradually rises in order to increase the cardiac output so as to maintain oxygenation of the vital centres. As the fetus has limited capacity of increasing the stroke volume, it increases its heart rate to maintain adequate cardiac output (Arulkumaran, 1992).

Baseline tachycardia is often the first clinical sign of fetal hypoxia (distress) on ordinary auscultation.

Infection

Both maternal and fetal infection may result in tachycardia as the temperature rises above 38°C/100.4°F. Hence, maternal temperature should be taken every two hours in labour specially in presence of fetal tachycardia and in the cases of prolonged labour. Often fetal tachycardia returns to normal when maternal fever is reduced (a vaginal probe which can measure the fetal temperature in labor is being designed).

Epidural analgesia

(See Chapter 24—'Role of CTG for Patients Getting Epidural Analgesia in Labor').

Pre-term fetus

As mentioned above, due to immaturity of the parasympathetic system pre-term fetus may manifest some tachycardia. Such a tachycardia may be considered physiological, provided that all potentially ominous aetiologies have been ruled out (also See Chapter 26—'Special Problems of CTG Monitoring of Preterm Pregnancy').

Drug treatment

Drugs used to arrest premature labour, e.g. the beta adrenergic agents like Salbutamol, Ritodrin, etc. can produce tachycardia because of excessive sympathetic activity.

Administration of Atropine to the mother has been shown to induce fetal tachycardia by vagolysis.

Anemia

Severe maternal and fetal anemias may result in baseline tachycardia. Fetal anaemia can occur in pregnancies complicated by hemolytic disease or fetal bleeding. Vasa-praevia, amniocentesis and anticoagulant therapy are some of the well known causes of fetal bleeding (Flynn and Kelly, 1982).

Cardiac failure

Maternal cardiac failure has been known to produce fetal baseline tachycardia (Flynn and Kelly, 1982).

Fetal heart tachyarrhythmia

Obviously, this would be associated with fetal tachycardia (Ingemarsson et al., 1993).

Degrees and Types of Tachycardia

- Mild—160–180 bpm
- Severe—Above 180 bpm
- If the rate exceeds 200 bpm the risk of fetal heart decompensation is very high.

Incidental Tachycardia

This short-term tachycardia is seen usually after a period of vigorous or prolonged fetal movement and is normal. In such instances baseline variability is not affected.

The above pattern is often seen after a period of 'quiet sleep' of fetus and as the fetus wakes up and makes lot of movement (**Fig. 12.3**).

Complicated Baseline Tachycardia

Any baseline tachycardia complicated by other untoward CTG features such as—loss of baseline variability and/or deceleration of any type (**Fig. 12.4**) is extremely ominous and call for fetal blood sampling and pH estimation or immediate delivery. This pattern is associated with *highest incidence of acidosis* (Steer, 1986). Late deceleration, which constitutes a strong evidence of fetal hypoxia, is seen more commonly with fetal tachycardia (also see examplary tracing in Chapter 13—**Figs 13.12** and **13.13**). ·

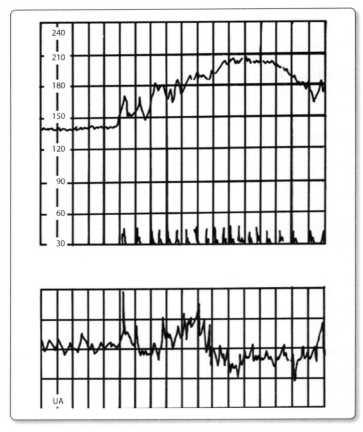

Fig. 12.3 This is an extreme, rather unusual, case of FM acceleration. Notice in the first part of the tracing—the baseline variability was almost nil (1–2 bpm) the fetus was probably in its quiet sleep. Suddenly the fetus woke up and started making vigorous movements causing such exceptional acceleration leading to actual tachycardia. Notice when heart rate reached 200 bpm the baseline variability flattened indicating some degree of temporary decompensation

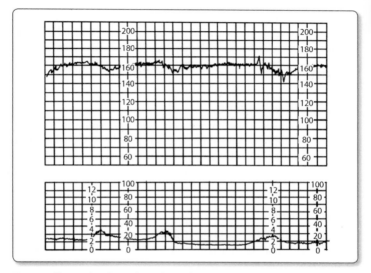

Fig. 12.4 Showing baseline tachycardia (160 bpm) with almost total loss of variability. Notice also the very shallow type II dips. This is a case of complicated baseline tachycardia and is ominous

BRADYCARDIA

Baseline bradycardia means sustained (not transient) decrease in FHR to below 120 bpm. Just as for baseline tachycardia, such label should be put on only after observing the tracing for *a minimum period of 10 minutes*.

Causes of Baseline Bradycardia
Hypoxemia

Fall in PO_2 in fetal blood stimulates chemoreceptors present in carotid and aortic bodies and causes baseline bradycardia.

Tissue Hypoxia

This develops as the hypoxia gets more severe and prolonged and causes more severe baseline bradycardia. Tissue hypoxia, which leads to metabolic acidosis, is responsible for this severity. In such cases in addition to baseline bradycardia, there also occurs reduced baseline variability and deceleration. It has been found that *fetal acidosis develops if bradycardia lasts for more than 20 mins.* (Ingemarsson, et al. 1993).

Local Anesthetic Agent

Bradycardia which is sometimes seen soon after epidural block or paracervical block (now very rarely used) may be due to the direct action of local anesthetic agents on fetal myocardium as the drug passes from mother to fetus. Such bradycardia usually does not last more than 20 minutes (Ingemarsson, et al. 1993).

Narcotic Drugs

These may reduce the baseline by 10–20 bpm perhaps due to reduction in fetal activity (Ingemarsson, et al. 1993). See **Figure 13.41** in Chapter 13.

Mild (Partial) Umbilical Cord Compression

Trapping of cord, e.g. between fetal limbs can also possibly cause temporary baseline bradycardia which usually gets corrected by itself as the fetus moves under the stress of the cardiovascular disturbance caused by partial compression. On turning the patient from one side to another (also) relieves such compression and consequent bradycardia (see early deceleration later). Such happenings are more common with oligohyramnios and postdated cases. Incidental tight stretching of the cord over fetal trunk can also cause such, more than transient, bradycardia.

Postdated Fetus (40 Plus Weeks)

According to Steer (1986), at this fetal age, rates between 100–120 bpm can be considered as normal provided there are no other abnormality. However, it is best in such cases to do a VAST (Vibroacoustic stimulation test) to double check that it is not due to hypoxia or odd short-term cord compression. These cases must be monitored very closely not by CTG alone but also by ultrasound, i.e. by Amniotic fluid index (AFI) and biophysical profile.

Head Compression

Persistent bradycardia specially in the second stage of labor in the range of 100–120 bpm has been reported to be associated with • occipito-posterior and • occipito-transverse position with very rare incidence of acidosis and almost invariable good neonatal outcome (Cunningham, et al. 1989). However, such bradycarida may happen late in labour even with normal presentation if the descent of the head through the birth canal is very rapid (Ingemarsson, et al. 1993).

This pressure related bradycardia is thought to be caused by sustained vagal centre stimulation resulting from raised intracranial pressure occasioned by mild fetal head compression.

Heart Block

Congenital atrioventricular block obviously would present as baseline bradycardia.

BASELINE VARIABILITY OF FHR

Definition

Normally, the baseline FHR is found to vary between 5–15 bpm every 10 to 20 seconds, i.e. at the frequency of 3–6 cycles per minute. This is called baseline variability. However, the minute irregularity that is invariably seen in the CTG trace line, which gives it a somewhat saw-toothed appearance and which represents the real beat-to-beat variation of FHR, is also referred as baseline variability (see short-term variability).

Mechanism of Its Occurrence

This has already been described earlier in this chapter. Basically, it has been found to be brought about by the constant interaction that goes on between sympathetic and parasympathetic nervous system of the fetus with ever changing relative dominance of one system over the other and *vice versa*.

Magnitudes of Variability and Their Significance
- Less than 5 bpm—Ominous
- Between 5–10 bpm—Normal but needs observation
- Between 10–20 bpm—Healthy fetus
  (Variability between 20–25 is also normal but not seen commonly)
- More than 25 bpm—Needs critical observation.

How to Find Out the Magnitude of Baseline Variability
The magnitude of baseline variability is to be found out by drawing a line each along the highest and the lowest projection of FHR trace *during one minute period* (**Fig. 12.5**).

Best Time to Assess Variability During Labor
In labor, the best time to assess the magnitude of variability is in between contractions so as to avoid confusion with the effect of contraction on FHR.

Physiological Explanation of Normal Variability
Presence of normal baseline variability indicates that, primarily, the neurological (autonomic) control mechanism of the fetal heart is intact and is working satisfactorily—the rare possibility of heart block being excluded.

However, the precise relationship between short-term and long-term variability is not quite clear yet. It has been suggested that while long-term variability is due to parasympathetic-sympathetic see-saw interaction, the short-term variability is possibly, primarily, the reflection of fluctuation within the parasympathetic system (Ingemarsson, et al. 1993).

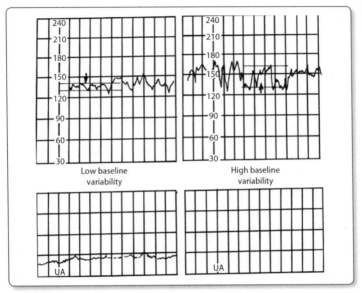

Fig. 12.5 Showing the method of precisely ascertaining the magnitude of baseline variability. A line each is to be drawn along the highest and the lowest projection of FHR trace

Causes of Changes in Baseline Variability
Hypoxia

It has been suggested that in conditions of chronic hypoxia, as the para-sympathetic control is lost first, which is mainly responsible for variability of FH, decreased variability results. If baseline variability is preserved but the tracing shows other abnormal features—it indicates that autonomic nervous system is not yet severely affected by the hypoxia and the fetus is trying to compensate (Arulkumaran, 1992).

Fetal Acidosis

This, almost invariably, results in reduced variability (less than 5 bpm) as can be confirmed by fetal blood sampling in laboring patients. However, only 50 per cent of cases with low variability lasting longer than 3 hours (180 mins) show fetal acidosis (Ingemarsson, et al. 1993). Low variability is also seen in CTG just before fetal death—the so called 'terminal pattern'. See in **Figure 13.46.**

In contrast, low FHR variability can sometimes be seen for several hours with good Apgar at birth. In such cases it is best to do fetal blood sampling or VAST to determine the real significance of low variability instead of prolonged monitoring and waiting in panic.

Prematurity

As explained below under long-term variability, low variability can be normal for fetuses under 34 weeks of gestation. These fetuses, due to immaturity of their cardiovascular system, are less able to increase their heart rate in response to changes in demand. Besides, these immature fetuses also, normally, have been found to exhibit small deceleration of FHR of about 15–20 bpm lasting for 10–20 seconds in absence of uterine contraction (Steer, 1986).

Fetal Sleep

This has been discussed in details in the exclusive chapter devoted on it (see Chapter 18—'Fetal Sleep, Rest, Activity and CTG').

Administration of CNS Depressant Drugs

Drugs like Diazepam, Pethidine, Magnesium sulphate, etc. administered to the mother reduce baseline variability of their fetus by the action of these on fetal CNS (see in **Fig. 13.41**).

Local Anesthetic Drugs

The 'caine' group of drugs are also well known to cause reduced variability.

Fetal CNS Abnormality

It's association with low variability has been observed. Before taking up these cases for Cesarean for fetal distress—it is recommended that an anomaly scan should be done.

Fetal Heart Malformation

It's association with low variability has often been observed. Here also, before taking up these cases for Cesarean for fetal distress—it is recommended that an anomaly scan should be done.

Baseline Tachycardia

Severe tachycardia (180+) is almost invariably associated with low variability (**Fig. 12.6**).

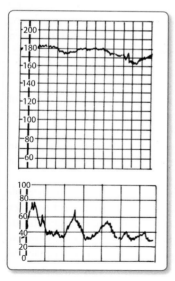

Fig. 12.6 Baseline tachycardia (it is 180 bpm here) is 'almost invariably associated with low variability (2–3 bpm here). Both are evidences of fetal hypoxia and decompensation

Types of Baseline Variability

Baseline variability has been classified into four types as follows:

- Short-term variability
- Long-term variability
- Sinusoidal pattern
- Wandering baseline

Short-term Variability

This signifies the variation in the interval between two beats of the heart which, in cardiotocographic context, means the interval between two R waves of fetal ECG (the R-R interval) as picked up through scalp electrode see **Figure 5.8** in Chapter 5. Short-term variability, being so minute, is a bit difficult to assess visually. What can be observed visually is blunting or exaggeration of the so-called teeth of the saw (**Fig. 12.7**). The only accurate way of quantitatively measuring it is by fetal ECG *with computer analysis*. FHR picked up externally by the ultrasonic transducer does not give the real short-term variability.

It is better seen on tracing done at higher paper speed, i.e. when the paper is run on at 3 cm/min speed rather than 1 cm/min speed.

Long-term Variability

This denotes the oscillatory changes that occur during the course of one minute in FH tracing, relative to it's baseline rate. Occurrence of 3-6 shifts is recognised as normal (**Fig. 12.8**).

Though by definition long-term variability is to be judged on one minute tracing, for proper interpretation, it is best observed for several minutes—*at least three minutes*.

Further, it is noteworthy that though ideally long-term variability has to be analysed both on the criterion of oscillation frequency (number of shifts per minute) and also on the factor of amplitude of variation, however, since oscillation frequency is a bit cumbersome and time consuming to find out from the tracing, for practical purposes, to judge the degree of variability, it is the amplitude of fluctuation, i.e. the *'band width'* which is analysed (**Fig. 12.8**).

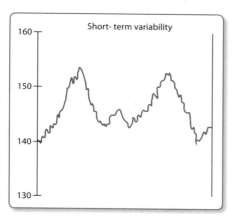

Fig. 12.7 Note the fine (not big waves) saw toothed appearance of the FHR tracing line. Each minute spike or tooth of the saw represents one heart beat and each of these is triggered by R wave of fetal ECG

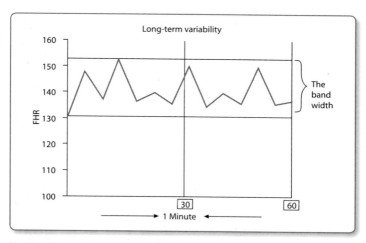

Fig. 12.8 Note the three parameter of baseline variability in the simulated drawing of long-term variability over one minute period. There occurred.
• 4 cycles of variation
• At intervals of 10–15 seconds
• Of amplitude between 10–15 bpm in relation to mean baseline

It has been found that with increasing gestational age both short-term and long-term variability increase. This occurs due to increasing vagal influence. This fact has to be specially remembered when monitoring cases of premature labour around 30–32 weeks in which case a finding of low variability may really be quite normal.

Sinusoidal Pattern

This is actually a relatively rare variety of long-term variability. In this the 'amplitude' and the 'period' of variation remains more or less *constant* giving the trace a smooth regular wavy appearance (see in **Figs 12.9** and **13.25**). In this pattern the amplitude of oscillations usually varies between 5–15 bpm.

Sinusoidal oscillations of more than 25 bpm is considered ominous.

Clinical correlation of sinusoidal pattern

1. The main underlying clinical cause of sinusoidal pattern has been found to be fetal anemia and consequent hypoxia as can be found in hemolytic disease of the fetus.

2. Massive fetal hemorrhage from whatever cause, e.g. maternal anti-coagulent therapy (Aspirin, Warfarin, etc.), bleeding vasapraevia, cordocentesis, etc. have also been found to be associated with sinusoidal pattern. The latter point has been proved experimentally in pregnant sheep. For clinical coroboration please see the tracing in Figure 13.4. It is from a case of severe fetal bleeding due to Aspirin therapy given to the mother as treatment of IUGR.

3. High FHR variability with somewhat regular pattern is also seen in some cases of cord compression during labour but this is better classed under variable deceleration (see later). See trace in **Figures 13.23 and 13.24** in Chapter No. 13.

4. Maternal administration of some sedative and analgesic drugs like Alphaprodine, Meperidin, Pethidine (reversible by administration of Naloxone) and Butaphanol have also been reported to induce this pattern of FHR (Cunningham, et al. 1989).

5. Transient sinusoidal rhythm has been reported even during normal labor (Cunningham, et al. 1989; Mishell, et al. 1993).

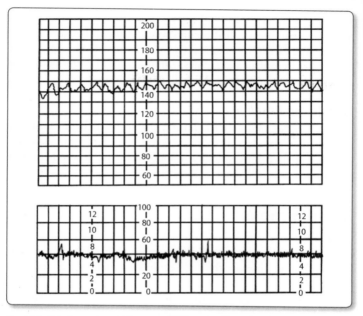

Fig. 12.9 This shows sinusoidal pattern of FHR tracing. Notice here the 'Amplitude' and 'Period' of variation of FHR is more or less consultant giving the trace a smooth regular wavy appearance

6. Sinusoid-like CTG pattern of short duration with preserved FM reactivity and variability has been correlated with rhythmic movements of fetal mouth (Ingemarsson, et al. 1993).

Subtypes of sinusoidal pattern

'TRUE'

'PSEUDO'.

'True' sinusoidal FHR pattern

It occurs with a frequency of 3 to 6 cycles per minute in a fixed long-term pattern *'alternating with smooth flat baseline intervals'* exhibiting a profound loss of beat-to-beat variability.

'Pseudo' sinusoidal FHR pattern

Sinusoidal pattern is called pseudo when in the in-between period the baseline variability is preserved—not flattened. This type of sinusoidal pattern which alternates with normal FH pattern does not carry ominous significance (Mishell, et al. 1993).

Wandering Baseline

This is a rather rare pattern. This is characterised by an unsteady baseline that "wanders" between 120 and 160 beats/min. Such pattern is suggestive of neurologically abnormal fetus. It is sometimes a preterminal event (William's Obstetrics, 2010).

ACCELERATIONS

Definition

From the baseline rate a sudden increase in FHR by more than 15 bpm lasting for more than 15 seconds is considered as acceleration (**Fig. 12.1**).

However, there are two criteria for measuring this 15 seconds—called short criterion and long criterion.

According to '**short criterion**' 15 seconds should be measured from the beginning of acceleration to return to baseline

According to '**long criterion**' it is the *'maintenance of FHR at 15 bpm acceleration level'* for 15 seconds which should be considered as qualifying.

However, a recent study has cleared this ambiguity about criteria. This study found that both the methods were of the same sensitivity and specificity. Hence, nowadays, the use of short criterion, which is more practical, is recommended (Arias 1993).

Cause

Primary Cause

FH acceleration almost invariably is caused by active fetal movement which may be palpable, sometimes visible over mother's abdomen, sometimes can be seen on uterine contraction tracing (as artefact) or may be verbally expressed by the mother on being asked or, while she is having her CTG, she would have marked them on the CTG tracing paper with the help of the remote event marker (patient button) which is given to her for the purpose. However, there are two exceptions to the above explanation.

a. FH acceleration may occur in absence of percieved movement by the mother.

b. Acceleration may not occur with every small movement that can be seen during ultrasonography.

Actocardiograph with automatic fetal movement monitoring facility is able to clear the above ambiguity.

Other Causes

- Uterine contraction
- Fetal stimulation

Acceleration coinciding with 'uterine contraction'

This phenomenon is called *periodic acceleration*. Two reasons have been ascribed to this:

a. Uterine contraction provokes fetal movement which in turn causes FH acceleration.

b. Acceleration may be an early sign of partial cord compression. In this specific situation FH acceleration is compensatory in nature and follows 'immediately' an episode of transient hypoxia' caused by cord compression during the contraction. As the degree of compression increases—this pattern gradually takes the shape of variable deceleration (see variable deceleration).

Acceleration in Response to 'Fetal' Stimulation

Incidental stimulation: This includes abdominal palpation and manipulation (like Version) and also vaginal fetal manipulation.

Incidental fetal stimulation may occur due to co-incidental fetal stimulation during the following vaginal procedures –

- Exploratory palpation for finding specially the position (of the occiput) of fetus in relation to pelvis
- During ARM (artificial rupture of membranes)
- During scalp electrode application
- During fetal blood sampling, etc.

    In each case the CTG tracing done during the procedure should show acceleration if the fetus is healthy.

Investigative stimulation: This includes -

- Vibro Acoustic stimulation (see later) and
- Scalp stimulation

    as a part of stimulation tests (see later).

Note: During an episode of fetal hyperactivity—the consequent repeated FM acceleration may merge into one another to raise the baseline FHR to above 160 bpm. If such a thing is detected during a CTG session monitoring should be continued until the baseline settles to normal (see **Fig. 12.3**).

Significance of Occurrence of Acceleration

Beard, et al. (1971) found that when FHR pattern exhibited accelerations the incidence of fetal acidosis was nil. Arulkumaran (1992) found that even in the presence of suspicious or abnormal traces, accelerations induced by external stimuli were indicative of a nonacidotic state, and this constitutes the basis of Vibroacoustic stimulation test—VAST (see trace in **Figs. 13.26** and **13.27**) and scalp stimulation test (see **Figs. 13.37** to **13.39**).

So, the overall conclusion is—presence of qualifying *acceleration signifies healthy state of the fetus.*

Though, as a corollary to above, absence of acceleration in a trace should be indicative of compromised state of the fetus but the position here is not very clear cut as with presence of acceleration. Hence, it is recommended that such cases should be monitored for longer period and be investigated further to arrive at a decision.

DECELERATIONS
Definition
From the baseline rate a sudden decrease in FHR by more than 15 bpm lasting for more than 15 seconds but less than two minutes is considered as deceleration (Ingemarsson, et al. 1993).

A Clever Definition of Deceleration
(**'Number of beats lost'** due to deceleration)

To make the definition more scientific and relevant, it has been suggested that the *'number of beats lost'* due to deceleration should also be taken into account in the definition so as to project the gravity of deceleration. In fact, newer CTG machines with automatic computer analysis facility, incorporates this parameter.

Objections in attaching too much importance to beat loss:

i. Shallow late deceleration, which are usually associated with intrauterine growth retardation, which may be seen in these cases even at early third trimester, would not receive their due importance through this parameter,

ii. Sharp and severe variable deceleration associated with cord compression, which is a very serious situation, does not always show that great degree of beat loss.

Significance
Contrary to what is true about acceleration, in any FHR tracing, deceleration whatever may be its type—should better be absent.

It is noteworthy that while during labor it is possible for some nonpathological type of deceleration to occur (see below), its occurrence during antenatal period should always be considered pathological.

Types
Classically, deceleration has been classified into three types as follows:
• Early deceleration

- Late deceleration
- Variable deceleration
  These have been discussed below.

Early Deceleration (Type I DIP)

Nomenclature

This is also called 'Synchronous deceleration' because it exactly synchronises with uterine contraction. The other term used for it is 'reflex deceleration' because here the bradycardia has been proved to be due to reflex stimulation of the vagal centre by the compression of the fetal head during contraction. A convincing evidence that it is so is the observation that this type of deceleration can be abolished by the vagolytic drug Atropine.

Classical Features (see Figs 12.10 and 13.9)

1. The dip in FHR is 'V' shaped with a 'sharp' lowest point.
2. The apex of V coincides with the peak (apex) of uterine contraction.
3. Deceleration starts very shortly after the beginning of contraction, hence it is called 'early'.
4. Deceleration recovers fully by the end of the contraction.
5. Deceleration is short lived.
6. Baseline FHR and baseline variability of FHR remain normal in between contraction.

Degree of Early Deceleration

Small — Depth of the dip is less than 40 bpm.
Large — Depth of the dip is more than 40 bpm.
        Rarely, the rate falls to below 100 bpm.

Causes of Early Deceleration

Head compression

Early deceleration indicates that patient is at the end of first stage or in second stage of labour with head deep in the pelvis which is getting compressed during contraction (see 'nomenclature' above).

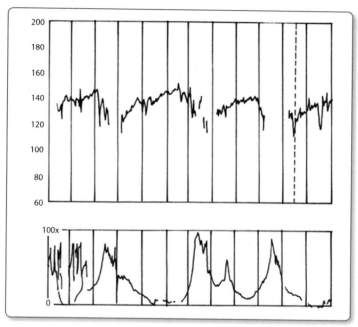

Fig. 12.10 This is a tracing of typical type I dip or early deceleration. Notice that the deceleration has 'started early' in contraction and recovered before the contraction is over. Also notice that the lowest point of deceleration has exactly coincided with the peak of uterine contraction. The important thing here is—the baseline FHR and baseline variability of FHR is preserved. This patient was fully dilated with head deep in the pelvis. Notice that the third dip was of greater magnitude than fast two dips. This was produced by finger pressure on head during PV during that particular contraction exaggerating the head compression and thereby aggravating the deceleration

Partial cord compression

This is how cord compression causes transient deceleration through mechanical stress: Cord compression—constriction of arterial outflow in the cord—damming back the fetal blood in its aorta—rise of blood pressure in aorta—triggering of stretch receptors in aorta—

stimulation of vagal center—slowing of heart (deceleration)—restoration of BP to normal (Steer, 1986).

Significance of Early Deceleration

Early deceleration, if 'uncomplicated', does not signify hypoxia or acidosis and hence immediate intervention is usually not necessary in these cases. However, it has been suggested that it is possible for coexistent mild hypoxia to potentiate the effect of early deceleration (Steer, 1986) when the pattern would gradually change into late deceleration shape (see **Fig. 13.10**). *Hence, tracing should be continued in these cases right upto delivery.*

The word 'uncomplicated' means absence of abnormality of baseline FH rate and baseline variability in the tracing in between the episodes of deceleration.

Note

There is one other thing to be remembered about decelerations in general—that during deceleration, due to reduction in heart rate, a significant proportion of cardiac output is lost which can lead to secondary hypoxia and acidosis (Steer,1986)—if the situation is allowed to prolong.

Management of Early Deceleration

a. A prompt vaginal examination is to be done:
   i.   To know the state of progress of labour (i.e. dilatation and descend),
   ii. To exclude any obstruction in the passage causing the compression,
   iii. To exclude cord prolapse.
b. Tracing must be continued to watch whether other ominous features are making their appearance or not, and one has to act accordingly.

LATE DECELERATION (TYPE II DIP)
Nomenclature

It is that type of 'contraction associated' deceleration of FHR which starts only *'late in contraction'* and does not return to normal baseline until after the contraction is over.

Occurrence of late deceleration on the face of artificially induced uterine contraction forms the basis of Contraction Stress Test (CST), Oxytocin Challenge Test (OCT) and Nipple Stimulation Stress Test (NSST) (see Chapter 15—'Applied Cardiotocography—Antenatal').

According to FIGO (1987)—there must be three or more late decelerations following 'consecutive' contractions for a diagnosis of late deceleration to be made.

Note

Late deceleration can occur even during antenatal period probably in response to Braxton-Hicks contractions. This may be seen in the cases of gross intrauterine growth retardation specially those which result from chronic placental insufficiency like those associated with long-standing pregnancy induced hypertension, recurrent small abruption of placenta, etc.

Classical Features

1. The dip in FHR trace is somewhat wide-mouthed 'U' shaped with round bottom.
2. The lowest point of 'U' does not coincide with the peak of uterine contraction. It comes after a 'time lag' of minimum of 15 seconds (see **Figs 12.11** and **13.5 to 13.8**).
3. Deceleration starts **'late'** in contraction and hence it is called late deceleration.
4. Deceleration does not recover by the end of the contraction. It outlasts the contraction.
5. Deceleration is much more prolonged than early deceleration.

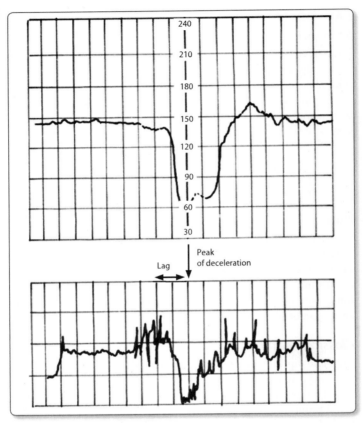

Fig. 12.11 This is a tracing of typical type II dip or late deceleration. Notice the deceleration has started 'late' in contraction and has outlasted the contraction. The time lag between the peak of deceleration and peak of contraction is evident. Note the compensatory acceleration at the end of deceleration. The other major ominous sign in this tracing is almost total absence of baseline variability

The Underlying Mechanism

Late deceleration always occurs due to hypoxia caused by uterine contraction resulting in reduced blood flow through the intervillous space the mechanism of which has been described in detail in the Chapter 17—'Applied Cardiotocography—Intranatal'. Given below are some of the important pathophysiological inter-relations of late deceleration which would help in the understanding of the underlying mechanism better:

a. *Relation with duration of contraction* It has been found that in late deceleration the degree of hypoxia produced is proportional to the 'duration of the contraction'—longer the contraction lasts greater is the chance of appearance of late deceleration. That is why sometimes late deceleration is not seen with every contraction, i.e. seen only with longer contraction and not with shorter contraction.

b. *Relation with amplitude of contraction* Besides above, it has also been shown that it is not just the duration—the amplitude of contraction is also important. Steer (1986) has shown that the degree of hypoxia was proportional to the duration of contraction 'above 30 mm of Hg' intra-amniotic pressure amplitude level.

c. *Relation with PO_2 of fetal blood* Steer (1986) has shown that late decelerations make their appearance only when the PO_2 in the fetus falls below 10 mm Hg. Deceleration is brought about by the effect of this severe 'hypoxaemia' on aortic and carotid chemoreceptors.

d. *Relation with pH level of fetal blood* The relation between late deceleration and pH level of fetal blood is not so direct. Only about 50% of fetuses showing late deceleration shows acidosis on fetal blood sampling. Animal experiments also have shown similar results.

e. *Probable relation with myocardial oxygenation* It has been concluded that it is the hypoxic depression of myocardium which is responsible for the late deceleration. This in turn causes reduced cardiac output and reduced ability of the fetus to respond to hypoxic situation like the uterine contraction.

f. *Relation with simple auscultation* If not interfered and the late deceleration is allowed to continue, the decelerations last longer and longer until one deceleration merges with the next. It is from this point that the bradycardia becomes discernible clinically on auscultation. By the time this happens fetus reaches the stage of 'tissue hypoxia' which ultimately leads to metabolic acidosis through anaerobic glycolysis with consequent lowering of pH of fetal blood.

g. *Role of vagus* In contrast to early deceleration, late deceleration cannot be abolished by the vagolytic drug Atropine (can only be modified). This excludes the role of vagus in its causation.

Degree of Late Deceleration

This can be classified in two ways as follows: (Ingemarsson, et al 1993)

a. Degree of drop in rate
   - Moderate—upto 100 bpm level
   - Severe—below 100 bpm level
b. Magnitude of beats lost
   - Less than 15 bpm
   - Between 15–45 bpm
   - Greater than 45 bpm

Prognostic Relation of Late Deceleration with Baseline Characters

This is an additional but a very important prognostic parameter. Here baseline character means—characters of tracing in between dips, i.e. during uterine quiescence. The prognostic relation in this context can be categorised as follows:

- Normal baseline rate and normal baseline variability in between— mild compromise.
- Abnormal baseline rate (tachycardia) and reduced baseline variability in between—severe compromise.

Clinical Causes of Late Deceleration

This can be classified into three groups as follows:

a. *Preuterine*
   - Maternal Hypotension

- Supine hypotension
- Following epidural block
  - Severe Anaemia
b. *Uterine*
  - Uterine Hyperactivity
    - Oxytocin Infusion given for induction or acceleration of labour
    - Prostaglandin induction
c. *Intrauterine*
  - Placental Insufficiency

This may be due to whatever cause, e.g. pregnancy induced hypertension, post dated pregnancy situation, APH, etc. IUGR is a frequent finding in this group.

Cause and Effect Relation

Of the above causes—in the first two groups the—cause being 'acute' and 'external' and the fetus being basically healthy—the fetal prognosis is usually very good, once the offending condition is detected and removed (See 'management' below). As it is done, late deceleration disappears promptly. In these cases, the baseline FHR and baseline variability remains normal in the in-between periods.

In the third group, because the fetus enters labor in already compromised state, even the constriction produced by the normal contractions of labor throws it out of balance and hence the causation of true hypoxic late deceleration in these cases. Since the condition is not reversible, as the time passes the situation gets worse. In these cases, in addition to late deceleration, baseline tachycardia and reduced baseline variability are usually seen in the periods between contractions.

Management

Intrauterine resuscitation

- **Turned on her side**—to relieve venacaval compression.
- **Stop uterine stimulent** drug if the patient has been on it like Oxytocin drip

- **Give tocolytic drug**—In case the contractions are too frequent and prolonged (even without oxytocin or Prostaglandin) one can do tocolysis by subcutaneous injection of Terbutalin 0.25 mg as a temporary measure while arranging for urgent operative delivery.
- *Additional advantages* of giving such beta receptor agonist (beta mimetic) drugs are—
    a. They oppose the increased vagal activity brought about by hypoxia and thereby reduce bradycardia and consequently *improve fetal cardiac output,*
    b. these also cause vasodilatation of placental vascular bed thereby *improving fetal blood flow* (Ingemarsson et al, 1993).
- **Oxygen inhalation** through mask at 10 litres/min.
- **Correct Hypovolaemia** where present (e.g. with epidural or in a grossly dehydrated patient as in a case of prolonged labor).
- **Elective Intravenous hydration:** 500 to 1000 ml of Ringer Lactate to be given over 20 minutes (William's Obstetrics, 2010).

By doing the above procedure deceleration will cease if the cause lay in these. But if deceleration continues in spite of above—one may assume that the causative factor is probably intrauterine (i.e. placental) in origin. However, to be doubly sure—one may do a Vibro acoustic stimulation test (VAST) and decide on the basis of its result as follows (see Chapter 19—'Vibroacoustic stimulation test by CTG'):

VAST reactive—one can wait with continuous monitoring

VAST non-reactive—Fetus should either be delivered immediately or it may be subjected to blood sampling and lactate or pH estimation if facility for this is available and if it can be done very expedeously—while arrangements are being made for prompt delivery.

Note

In the cases showing occasional late deceleration—if, in between contractions, the baseline FHR remains normal, baseline variability remains good and, specially, if FH accelerations are present—one can wait with the fetal monitor continuously working on the patient.

Variable Deceleration
Nomenclature

Variable deceleration means decelerations which are variable in their relation to uterine contraction which means:

- May come (variably) during any phase of contraction—not typically 'early' or 'late'.
- May or may not come with each and every contraction.

However, one can bring another connotation to the term variable, i.e. variability in the shape of the dip that the decelerations produce on the paper. Given the above, still the basic shape of the trace is usually found to be more or less like that of the letter 'M' (Steer, 1986) with minor departures (see **Figs 13.20 to 13.24**).

Besides above, decelerations also usually vary in degree of fall of FHR and also in their duration.

However, these decelerations have not been found to be related to the intensity of uterine contraction.

Typically variable decelerations are *short and sharp episodes* characterised by 'abrupt fall in FHR followed by rapid return to baseline'.

Etiology

The main cause

Variable deceleration has been thought to reflect a recurrent threat of decreased perfusion of the fetus arising from a ***disturbance in blood flow through the umbilical cord*** due to it's compression of varying degrees. This fact has been demonstrated through animal experiment and by Doppler velocimetry in human fetus. On Doppler examination, cord-compression has been found to cause the end-diastolic blood flow through the umbilical artery—to be abolished or even reversed.

Since in this abnormality both deceleration and return of FHR to baseline occur so abruptly the process has been thought to be of reflex nature. That the reflex is *of vagal origin* is proved by the fact that injection of atropine can abolish it.

The course of vascular events in variable deceleration has been described by Steer (1986) as follows:

a. *Events in the earlier (milder) stages of cord compression* Here, only the venous flow (being thin walled) is obstructed which leads to decreased venous return to fetal heart—a situation in which heart responds by producing compensatory tachycardia in order to maintain the blood pressure. This spurt of tachycardia explains the first peak of the 'M' shape of the tracing (see above).

b. *Events in later (more severe) stages of cord compressions* In this stage arterial blood flow is also obstructed leading to increased peripheral resistance and rise of blood pressure. Rise of blood pressure activates the aortic stretch receptors which in turn leads to activation of vagal centre in the brain producing bradycardia—and it is how the fetus attempts to restore its blood pressure to normal level. This explains the middle dipped portion of the 'M'.

The second peak of 'M' is caused by reactive tachycardia once the occlusion of cord was over.

In summary the ***typical 'M' shaped tracing*** of variable deceleration is formed by 'an acceleration before and an acceleration after'—a deep deceleration.

The other causes
• Rapid descend of fetal head through birth canal.
• Fetal head compression in normal second stage of labour.

In these two conditions the FH variability in between episodes of decelerations remain quite normal (Ingemarrson, et al 1993).

Predisposing Factors

Length of the cord

Both short cord (less than 35 cm) and long cord (more than 80 cm) have been found to be associated with higher incidence of variable deceleration (Ingemarrson, et al 1993). With short cord there is higher risk of cord-stretching and with long cord there is higher chance of entrapment. Cord round the neck or body of the fetus, if not stretched or compressed, does not give rise to variable deceleration.

Volume of liquor

Obviously with oligo-hydramnios there is higher chance of cord compression as can be seen in some cases of post-maturity. This, in fact, is the basis of giving amnioinfusion in these cases.

Deficiency of Wharton's jelly

This can happen with IUGR. (Ingmarsson, et al 1993). Here, due to loss of buffering action, cord is more likely to be compressed.

Breech presentation

It is well known that breeches carry higher risk of cord compression with the fetal thighs pressing on the cord during cotractions.

Occipito-posterior position

Higher incidence of variable deceleration has been reported with this presentation (Ingemarrson, et al 1993).

Face presentation

This also has been reported to show higher incidence of variable deceleration, possibly, due to compression of eyes (Ingemarrson, et al 1993).

Degree of variable deceleration

Depending on the magnitude of the dip, variable deceleration can be graded into three degrees as follows:

Mild	—	Drop upto 80 bpm level
Moderate	—	Drop upto 70 bpm level
Severe	—	Drop to lower level than 70 bpm

However, this grading has not been found to correlate well with Apgar score.

Prognosis of Variable Deceleration

It is not easy to give prediction on variable deceleration because while in some cases even after hours of such deceleration baby may be born with good Apgar, in some other cases fetus may become acidotic quite quickly. However, the following points should be given due consideration before taking decision:

Frequency of deceleration

If deceleration comes in very quick succession—not allowing the fetus to recover—risk of hypoxia is high.

Duration of deceleration

Longer the deceleration lasts—higher is the risk of hypoxia due to beat loss.

Shape of deceleration

This actually depicts the duration of deceleration. 'V shaped dips are short duration dips and hence carries almost no risk. But the 'U'—shaped dips which are long duration dips naturally carry higher risk of hypoxia.

Presence of initial acceleration

As usual (see acceleration), this is a reassuring sign about absence of acidosis. Actually, this initial acceleration may be viewed as if the fetus was going to accelerate in response to contraction but was interrupted by the vagal response to cord compression—bringing in the deceleration.

Rebound tachycardia

This means exaggeration of second peak of 'M'. It is not the same as the momentary acceleration that occurs at the end of each deceleration as the pressure from the cord gets released—it is an 'overshoot' and that's what matters. If at the end of each deceleration the baseline settles at a higher level (going towards baseline tachycardia), it should be considered as a sign of approaching hypoxia.

FHR pattern in between the episodes of variable deceleration

Baseline FHR is often difficult to assess with variable deceleration specially where the dips are too frequent with hardly any time for recovery (but frequent dips are serious in any case). Anyway, any element of baseline tachycardia present should be considered ominous.

Again, as already described, flattening of baseline variability is always a sign of hypoxia. In fact, absence of variability even during deceleration carries serious significance.

Mixed pattern

If variable deceleration shows an element of late deceleration specially with 'U' shaped bottom—it should be taken as a sign of hypoxia.

To summarise

Typically 'V shaped deceleration with mild degree of drop (not below 80 bpm level), not lasting more than 1 min., with normal baseline FHR and good variablity—usually do not make the baby hypoxic. However, these fetuses need constant monitoring to detect appearance of any untoward feature.

Variable deceleration with any other abnormal feature (see prognosis) carries the possibility of hypoxia or impending hypoxia.

Note

Actual cord prolapse, where cord gets directly and severly compressed due to absent bag of membranes—gives most severe form of prolonged and profound bradycardia and should be **urgently acted upon (delivered)**. *No time should be wasted in analysing the tracing.*

Management of Variable Deceleration

Positioning

It is a common experience that change of maternal position causes variable deceleration to disappear by, presumably, relieving the cord compression. So, the patient should be immediately turned to her left side—if that does not work-to her right side and if that does not work—even the knee-chest position may be tried.

Oxygen inhalation

Even though not all cases of variable deceleration signify hypoxia, to be on the safe side oxygen must be given because, after all, beat loss reduces the fetal cardiac output and turnover of fetal blood through the placenta.

Continuous monitoring and analysis of tracing

This will guide whether the patient should be delivered immediately or not based on the finding whether the tracing is becoming normal or more abnormal, i.e. turning into typical late deceleration pattern.

Tocolysis

This may be helpful by causing reduction in the intensity of contraction so that compression is relieved (see 'Late deceleration').

Amnioinfusion

As oligohydramnios, because of its potential to cause cord compression, is a very important predisposing and associated factor for variable deceleration hence the role of amnio-infusion. In fact, amnioinfusion has been shown to reduce—even make the deceleration disappear. This should be done through intrauterine pressure catheter after the rupture of the membranes. Warm normal saline at the rate of 10 to 15 ml/min. should be infused until the deceleration has disappeared. A maximum of 600 to 800 ml may be given.

Fetal blood sampling (FBS)

This is not indicated for severe cases (see prognosis) who should be delivered immediately. Mild cases may be observed by CTG alone. So, as it would appear from the above exclusions, it is really indicated in the cases of moderate degree only specially where normal delivery is not likely to occur soon to see whether more time can be allowed or not. Continuous CTG monitoring with F-ECG cum STAN would be a better option here than FBS.

Combined Deceleration
Definition

As the term implies, when a CTG tracing show's more than one type of deceleration it is called combined deceleration. It can be of two types:

▶ Early + Late deceleration

or

▶ Variable + Late deceleration

In fact, it is really the 'superimposition of late deceleration' is what matters in these cases because this constitutes definite evidence of hypoxia.

Shape

There is no typical shape. Occurrence of double dip in one contraction—giving the shape of the letter "W" (Ingemarsson et al, 1993) is what is to be looked for.

Cause

Ingemarsson et al (1993) found highest association of this type of tracing with oxytocin overstimulation. However, it can also happen with spontaneous labor.

Significance

It is same as late deceleration, i.e. indicates fetal hypoxic state.

Management

The first thing to do is to reduce or stop oxytocin drip if the patient has been on it.

The rest of the mangement will be same as that for late deceleration.

(Also see Chapter 17—'Applied Cardiotocography—Intranatal—the heading—

'Some unusual causes of deceleration during labor').

FORMULA OF 15 FOR CTG INTERPRETATION

For Acceleration

- FHR should rise by at least 15 bpm from baseline
- Acceleration should last at least for 15 seconds
- At least one such acceleration should occur during a 15 minutes period

For Deceleration

- FHR should drop by at least 15 bpm from baseline
- Dip should last for at least 15 seconds
- To call a deceleration "Late deceleration" the "Lag period" between lowest point of bradycardia and the peak of uterine contraction must be of at least 15 seconds duration.

ABNORMAL FHR TRACING ➡ TO ➡ ACIDOSIS INTERVAL

Fleischer et al (1982), demonstrated that with an averagely grown fetus at term with clear amniotic fluid, 50% of fetuses took the following time duration to become acidiotic after an abnormal or suspicious trace:

With repeated late decelerations	–	115 min (2 hours)
With repeated variable deceleration	–	145 min (2 1/2 hours)
With flat trace– (baseline variability of less than 5 bpm)		185 min (3 hours)

TRACING CHARACTER SEQUENCE AND DEGREE OF HYPOXIA

Normal trace
⬇

Early hypoxia	– Disappearance of acceleration with FM
	– Disappearance of acceleration with uterine contraction

⬇

Further hypoxia – Rising baseline FHR—baseline tachycardia

⬇

Further hypoxia – Reduction in baseline variability to less than 5 bpm, i.e. almost straight line CTG

⬇

Further hypoxia – Late deceleration with Braxton-Hicks contraction or labour contraction (Arulkumaran, 1992, Debdas, 1993)

FURTHER READING

1. Arias E. Practical guide to high-risk pregnancy and delivery, 2nd edition, Mosby Year Book, St Louis, 1993;3-20, 301–8 and 413–29.
2. Arulkumarn S. Obstetrics and Gynaecology for postgraduates, 1st edition, edited by Ratnam SS, Bhaskar Rao, K and Arulkumaran S, Orient Longman, Chennai, India, 1992;115–26.
3. Beard RW, Filshie GM, Knight CA, Roberts GM. J Obstet Gynaecol Br C With, 1971;78:865–81.
4. Debdas AK. Practical Cardiotocography, Published by Fetal Monitoring Research Centre, Jamshedpur, 1993;56–74.
5. FIGO. "Guidelines for the use of fetal monitoring" Int J Obstet Gynecol 1993;25:159–67.
6. Fleischer A, Schulman H, Jagani N, Mitchell J, Randolph G. Am J Obstet Gynecol 1982;144:55–60.
7. Flynn AM, Kelly J. Recent Advances in Obst and Gynae, Edited By John Bonnar, Vol-14, Churchill Livingstone 1982;25–45.
8. Fraser DM and Cooper MA in Myles Textbook for Midwives, 15th Edition, Monitoring the Fetus, Churchill Livingstone, London, 2009;481–4,
9. Ingemarsson I, Ingemersson E, Spencer JAD. Fetal heart rate monitoring a practical guide, Oxford University Press, Oxford, 1993;283–85.
10. Magowan B, Owen P, Drife J: Clinical Obst Gynae, 2nd edition, Monitoring the Fetus in labor, Elsevier, Edinburg, 2009;331–43.
11 Mishell DR, Kirschbaum TH, Morrow CP. Year Book of Obstetrics and Gynaecology-1993. Edited by these authors, Year book publisher, Chicago, 1993;136–62.
12. NICE (National Institute for Clinical Excellance) Guideline :The use of Electronic fetal monitoring: the use and interpretation of Cardiotocography in Intrapartum Fetal Surveillance, London, 2001
13. NICE (National Institute for Clinical Excellance) Guideline :The Clinical Guideline No. 70, Induction of labour, RCOG press, London, 2008
14. Steer PJ. Fetal heart rate patterns and their clinical interpretations, Oxford Sonicaid Ltd, Sussex, UK, 1986;1–44.
15. William's Obstetrics: 23rd Edition, Edited by Cunningham FG, Leveno KJ, Bloom SL, Hauth JC, Rouse DJ and Spong CY, Intrapartum Assessment, Mc Graw Hill, New York, 2010;410-43

CTG Interpretation—Examples of Tracings and Analysis— 'CTG Made Easy'

This chapter has been planned with a 'on the spot' obstetrician in view faced with a particular clinical situation and a tracing from that case. The object is to help the obstetrician to take the right decision. Almost all types of typical tracings have been presented here so that one can use one's CTG machine with great ease and confidence.

LIST OF TRACINGS PRESENTED

1. Non-reactive non-stress test (NST).
2. Reactive non-stress test.
3. Flat CTG.
4. Absolutely inert VAST-fetal hemorrhage.
5. Late deceleration with baseline tachycardia.
6. Shallow but prolonged late deceleration.
7. Deep type II dip.
8. Degrees of late deceleration.
9. Type I dip/early deceleration.
10. Combined decelerations (early + late).
11. Peculiarities of CTG tracing of second stage of labour done through external technique.
12. Complicated baseline tachycardia.
13. Complicated baseline tachycardia.
14. Oxytocin induced profound bradycardia.
15. Hyperstimulation by oxytocin.

16. Nipple stimulation stress test.
17. FHR response to Hyperstimulation of uterus.
18. Active awake fetus.
19. Deceleration with fetal movement.
20. Variable deceleration.
21. Variable deceleration.
22. Variable deceleration-follow up.
23. Variable deceleration.
24. Variable deceleration due to head compression in second stage of labour.
25. Sinusoidal pattern.
26. Fetal Vibroacoustic stimulation test (VAST).
27. Fetal Vibroacoustic stimulation test.
28. Atypical-spiky VAST.
29. Atypical-spiky VAST.
30. An unusal response to VAST.
31. Biphasic VAST.
32. Episodes of deceleration.
33. Progressive baseline bradycardia.
34. Atypical acceleration with contraction.
35. Uterine polysystole.
36. Admission test.
37. Scalp stimulation test.
38. Scalp stimulation test.
39. Scalp stimulation test.
40. Effect of Pethidine on FHR tracing.
41. Effect of Diazepam on FHR tracing.
42. Iatrogenic CTG abnormalities.
43. CTG characteristics of pre-term pregnancy.
44. CTG characteristics of pre-term pregnancy.
45. Sequence of FHR pattern from fetal distress to fetal death.
46. Terminal FHR pattern.
47. False fetal distress.
48. False fetal distress.
49. Fetal actocardiograph.
50. Biophysical profile by actocardiography.

A Non-Reactive 'Non-Stress Test' (NST) (Fig. 13.1)

This is a 'non-reactive' antenatal CTG tracing showing absence of acceleration of FH with fetal movement over 20 minutes period which is the standard duration for performing NST. Baseline FHR is normal here but the baseline variability is less than 5 bpm which is worrying.

Though 'non-reactive' NSTs are recognised sign of fetal compromise since it has about 50% false-positive rate these patients need further observation (between 45 to maximum 60 minutes period—See Chapter 12—'CTG Interpretation—Theoretical Considerations') and investigations like VAST or biophysical profile assessment.

Additionally, also note two gaps in the FHR tracing—one just after the second FM mark and one just above the fourth FM marking. These are episodes of deceleration with FM. Please note that in the cases of such sudden interruption in FH tracing one must carefully see and ensure that it is not due to momentary dislocation of the transducer

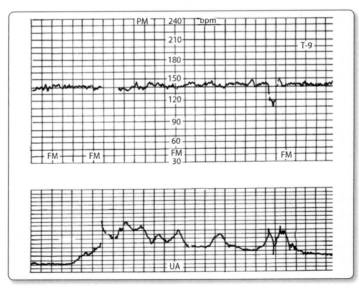

Fig. 13.1 Non-reactive non-stress test (NST)

due to maternal movement or any other external cause. Since this was an antenatal case both FH and uterine activity were recorded externally.

A Reactive Non-Stress Test (Fig. 13.2)

This is a ten minutes tracing from an uncomplicated case who had a routine NST for fetal monitoring because she was postdated by two days. Four clear qualifying reactivity (accelerations) are seen—of at least 15 bpm magnitude and of at least 15 seconds duration. Baseline FHR is around 130 bpm and baseline variability is between 5–10 bpm. The pointed dark vertical lines of about 1 cm length each at the

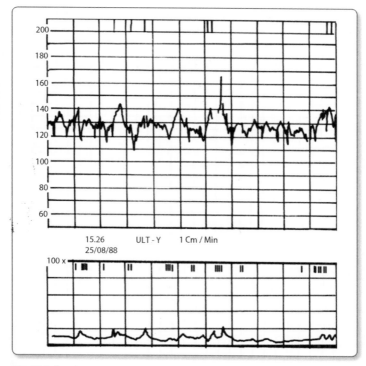

Fig. 13.2 Reactive non-stress test

very top of the tracing paper denote the number of fetal movement as registered by the mother through the remote event marker (Patient button). The series of very tiny dark lines near the top margin of the toco segment of the paper are the automatic annotations of the occurrence of fetal movement and is done by the 'acto' part of the CTG machine. Notice that the episodes of FH accelerations have more or less coincided with fetal movement marks which is the key point here. Compare this tracing with the immediately previous tracing (**Fig. 13.1**) and notice the drastic difference.

Flat CTG (Fig. 13.3)

This is a typical tracing of poor baseline variability (i.e. poor beat-to-beat variation) also called 'Flat' tracing. The variability here would be

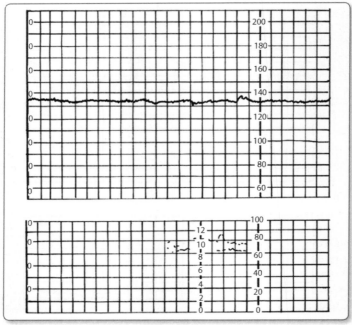

Fig. 13.3 Flat CTG

something like 1 or 2-bpm whereas minimum acceptable is 5-bpm-normal range being 10-15 upto 25 bpm. This is an antenatal CTG tracing of a case of gross IUGR with diminished FM at 37th week. The patient had not been on any sedation. The tracing was continued for over 90 minutes but variability did not increase and no fetal movement was registered by mother during the period. Even manual stimulation of fetus by abdominal palpation did not have any effect on FHR. So, a caesarean section was done because such prolonged and grossly diminished variability is often associated with fetal hypoxia and acidosis. A 2.1 kg baby was delivered with Apgar 4 at 1 min. Liquor was very scanty and thick though not meconium stained. Without the use of CTG such fine kind of FHR abnormality cannot be diagnosed since the baseline FHR, which is the only thing that can be appreciated by fetoscope or Doptone, would always have been found to be normal-around 138-bpm (see tracing) on auscultation in such a case. Ideally such cases should have double checking of FHR response by applying Vibroacoustic stimulation to exclude the rare event of prolonged fetal sleep. Fetal CNS abnormality should also be kept in mind. A biophysical profile is also a good proposition in such a case. If the facility was available—a Doppler blood flow study would have made the position even clearer.

Absolutely Inert VAST-Fetal Hemorrhage (Fig. 13.4)

Primi, 30 years, IUGR at 34 weeks, normotensive, had been on low dose Aspirin therapy, came with the complaint of sudden cessation of FM. CTG showed baseline of 150 with very poor (1–2) variability. There was no response to 3 consecutive Vibroacoustic stimuli of 3 seconds duration each given at 3 minutes intervals. No FM was felt by the mother at any stage. In fact, an element of 'sinusoidal pattern' appeared after the third stimulus. Note a prolonged (3 mins) spontaneous deceleration at the beginning of tracing. VAST was repeated 3 times in next 12 hours with no response. So emergency cesarean was done. Baby's hemoglobin was only 3 GM. Baby died after about 6 hours in spite of blood transfusion. It was a case of fetal hemorrhage due to Aspirin therapy.

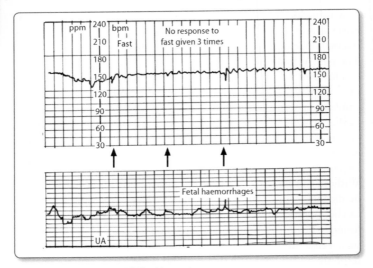

Fig. 13.4 Absolutely inert VAST-fetal hemorrhage

Late Deceleration with Baseline Tachycardia (Fig. 13.5)

Note that each deceleration has commenced late in contraction and has reached their lowest point only after a lag period of 45 seconds following the peak uterine contraction (paper speed—1 cm/min, FH and uterine activity were both recorded by external abdominal transducer). Notice the baseline tachycardia (160/min). This tallies with the common experience that late deceleration are commonly associated with baseline tachycardia. Such association is considered as an evidence of compensation on the part of the fetus to mitigate the hypoxic threat by increasing its heart rate. Also notice the flattening (less than 5 bpm) of baseline variability. So, this is an ominous tracing from three angles. This multigravida delivered normally in one hour ten minutes. Apgar was four at one minute.

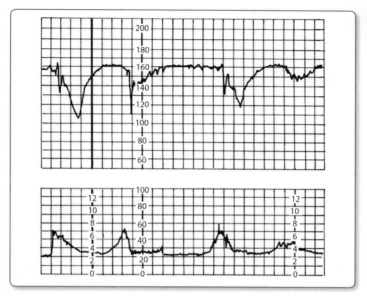

Fig. 13.5 Late deceleration with baseline tachycardia

Shallow but Prolonged Late Deceleration (Fig. 13.6)

Here is one more tracing of late deceleration or type II dip. Notice the late onset of deceleration, the long lag time and late recovery. There is also gross flattening of baseline variability (less than 5 bpm) but the baseline FHR is under 150. Patient delivered normally in next one and a half hour with Apgar 3 at one minute. Birth weight was 2.4 kg at 41 weeks and liquor was clear.

Deep Type II Dip (Fig. 13.7)

This 26 years old primi was a case of compensated mitral stenosis but was growth retarded by 4 weeks. CTG done in early labor showed deep late decelerations down upto 70 bpm. An emergency cesarean

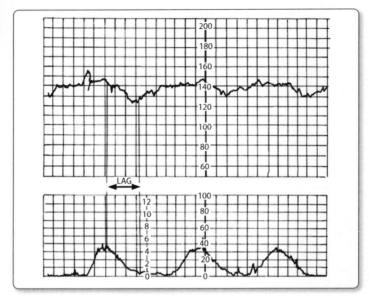

Fig. 13.6 Shallow but prolonged late deceleration

was done. Apgar was ten at one minute. Note, though baseline FHR was around 150 bpm, the baseline variability turned poor after the deceleration (this feature is noticeable only after the first dip).

Degrees of Late Deceleration (Fig. 13.8)

This tracing shows a series of five late decelerations within a period of fourteen minutes. Of these the first two were very deep-down to 100 bpm (drop by 80 bpm) and the next three were rather shallow-down by only 20 bpm. Obviously, the number of beats lost is much more in first two dips, than in subsequent three-duration of deceleration being more or less same in all three (around two minutes). Presence of baseline tachycardia (180 bpm) and almost total absence of variability make the case a critical one. An emergency cesarean section was done. The Apgar was four.

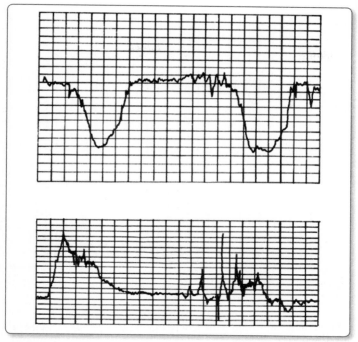

Fig. 13.7 Deep type II dip

Type I Dip/Early Deceleration (Fig. 13.9)

Notice the 3 classical features of early deceleration or type I dip namely-'early' start of deceleration right from the beginning of contraction, the precise coincidence of peak of contraction with the peak of deceleration and the recovery of FHR to normal pre-deceleration level by the end of contraction. Also notice in the tracing that baseline variability of FHR is well-maintained throughout the tracing indicating thereby good fetal oxygenation. Type I dip has been proved to be due to head compression and is almost always innocuous (see the immediately previous chapter, i.e. Chapter 12).

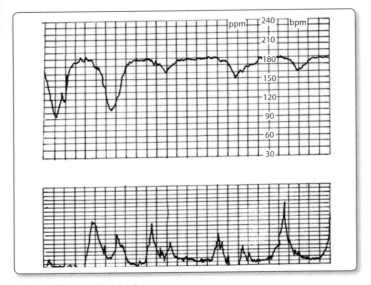

Fig. 13.8 Degrees of late deceleration

This patient was towards the end of first stage of labour (9 cm) with head at plus 2 cm level. She delivered normally 1 hour 50 minutes later with Apgar 10.

Combined Decelerations (Early and Late) (Fig. 13.10)

This tracing shows element of both early and late deceleration. Note, the late onset of dips and the invariable lag period which fits in well with the criteria of late deceleration. However, notice that the shape of the dips are not typical of type II. They are rather pointed and deep and of the shape of 'V' rather than of (round bottom) 'U'—a shape which is usual for dips of late deceleration. In this case, labor was augmented by oxytoxin drip and contraction frequency here, as can be seen on the chart, is four per ten minutes. This patient was almost fully dilated which brought in the element of head compres-

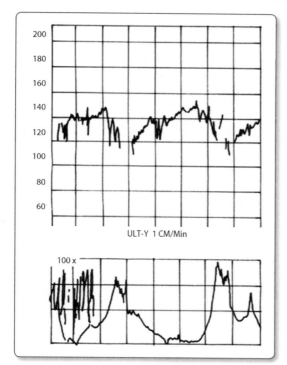

Fig. 13.9 Type I dip/early deceleration

sion in these dips and head compression is known to be the causative factor for early deceleration.

Peculiarities of CTG Tracing of Second Stage of Labor
Done through external technique (Fig. 13.11)

This tracing was taken just 15 mins. before delivery obtained through ultrasonic FH transducer and external toco transducer. The two features that are peculiar in this chart paper are:

a.   Intermittent discontinuity of FH tracing—This is due to loss of transducer-contact during pushing effort and maternal restlessness.

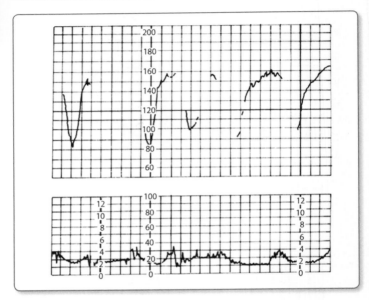

Fig. 13.10 Combined decelerations (early + late)

b. Saw-toothed appearance of uterine contraction tracing—This is
    due to maternal hyperbreathing. These disturbances are not seen
    when monitoring is done by internal method by the use of scalp
    electrode and intrauterine catheter.

Note: She had been contracting at the rate of one in every two and
half minutes and each contraction had been lasting for about forty five
seconds (paper speed 2 cm per min). Also note the type II element in
this tracing. In fact, there is also an element of variable deceleration in
the tracing. Short-term baseline variability is also poor (read Chapter
12 – " CTG Interpretation – Theoretical Considerations").

Complicated Baseline Tachycardia (Fig. 13.12)

This is a tracing of baseline tachycardia of about 180 bpm from a
patient in labor. However, this is not a case of simple baseline FHR

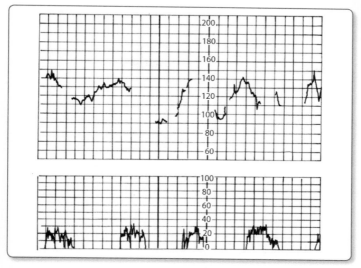

Fig. 13.11 Peculiarities of CTG tracing of second stage of labor done through external technique

abnormality as it may appear on first look. In addition to tachycardia there are two other subtle FHR abnormality in this tracing namely poor baseline variability (less than 5 bpm) and an episode of long deceleration lasting for about four minutes of the amplitude of 20 bpm. Such cases of complicated baseline tachycardia are well known to be extremely ominous and should be acted upon. If facilities are available fetal blood sampling and pH estimation is indicated. Of course simpler would be application of FECG with STAN. Unfortunately, in this tracing the important relation of bradycardia with contraction cannot be established because the latter has not been traced here. Maternal temperature in this case was 98.6° F and maternal pulse was 94 per min. These two parameters must be checked in every case of baseline tachycardia. This patient was delivered by cesarean section and Apgar was three.

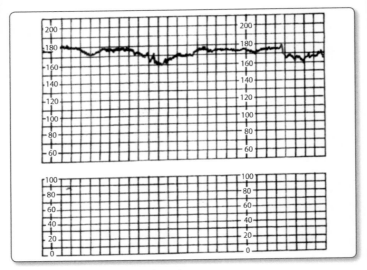

Fig. 13.12 Complicated baseline tachycardia

Complicated Baseline Tachycardia (Fig. 13.13)

Primi, 22 years at 39+ weeks was induced by ARM and oxytocin for pregnancy induced hypertension. It is obvious on the tracing that there is baseline tachycardia (160+). As regards variability, though the short term variability is grossly reduced (blunting of saw-tooth) the long term variability is maintained. After a short while the tracing started showing typical type II dips (not shown here). An emergency cesarean was done. Apgar was two at one minute and eight at five minutes. Birth weight was 3.4 kg.

Oxytocin induced Profound Bradycardia (Fig. 13.14)

In an otherwise normal second gravida labor was induced at term plus 8 days by ARM plus oxytocin. Soon after the oxytocin drip was started the toco trace showed tonic contraction and FH trace showed progressive bradycardia down to 60 bpm. Although the drip

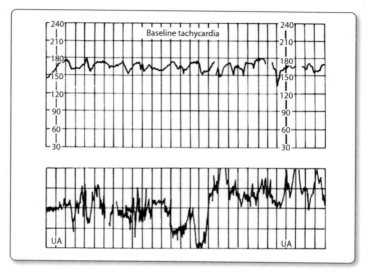

Fig. 13.13 Complicated baseline tachycardia

was stopped as soon as the FHR dropped to 90 bpm—recovery was delayed. At the end of bradycardia there was some compensatory tachycardia with a flat baseline. It is also clearly noticeable in the tracing that though for the first three minutes of deceleration, the variability was preserved the rest of the dip showed almost total loss of baseline variability. Patient had a normal delivery eight hours later without oxytocin with no other FH problem. Liquor was clear and Apgar was ten at one minute.

Hyperstimulation by Oxytocin (Fig. 13.15)

This tracing has been presented to show clonic uterine contraction, i.e. series of contraction in a row with very little or no relaxation in between as opposed to the tonic contraction. This has been brought about by oxytocin. This is in contrast to **Figure 13.14** where oxytocin had induced tonic contraction of uterus. Severe fetal hypoxia,

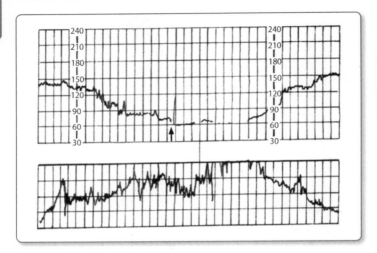

Fig. 13.14 Oxytocin induced profound bradycardia

as evidenced by severe prolonged bradycardia, is evident on the tracing. Note FHR recovered promptly on omission of oxytocin. Note also the post recovery compensatory tachycardia with almost total absence of variability which indicates that the fetus was still in hypoxic state.

Nipple Stimulation Stress Test (Fig. 13.16)

This is an old tracing of 1985. In this case, who was postdated by one week, contraction stress test was done by bilateral self-stimulation of nipple. This caused prolonged tonic contraction of the uterus which, in turn, brought about prolonged and profound deceleration of FH presumably due to hypoxia caused by occlusion of retroplacental vessels by the contracting uterus. This patient ultimately needed cesarean section when baby was found to have inhaled meconium. The Apgar was only three. Since we have had several such instances of hyperstimulation of uterus with nipple stimulation—we have abandoned this crude test.

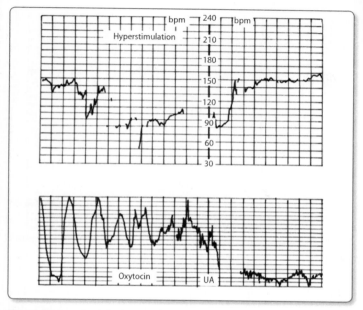

Fig. 13.15 Hyperstimulation by oxytocin

FHR Response to Hyperstimulation of Uterus (Fig. 13.17)

This tracing shows the effect of hyperstimulation of uterus on FHR. Here the hyperstimulation was caused by nipple stimulation (self) as a part of 'Nipple stimulation stress test'. In the toco channel, note the occurrence of series of contractions with almost no relaxation in between. The patient was a young normotensive primigravida postdated by eight days. Obviously, here hypoxia caused by prolonged successive uterine contractions has led to this profound prolonged bradycardia. Note in the last bit of tracing the compensatory tachycardia that occurred once the contraction eased and intervillous circulation improved. Notice that the baseline variability was almost nil in the whole FHR tracing. The patient was

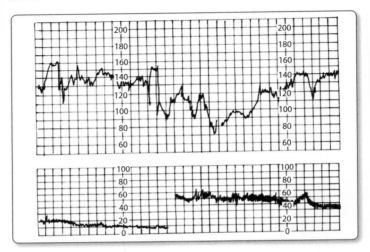

Fig. 13.16 Nipple stimulation stress test

delivered by cesarean section since the cervix was very unripe. The baby was found to have passed meconium and also had aspirated it. Apgar was three.

Active Awake Fetus (Fig. 13.18)

This is an antenatal non-stressed tracing. On first look there may be some confusion regarding the baseline FHR in this tracing. Please observe that it is lower FHR tracing, i.e. the rate between 120 and 130 bpm which is the actual baseline FHR. The humps which have arisen from this baseline are, in fact, large accelerations (by 30–35 bpm) due to vigorous fetal movements as recorded on the chart by the machine and as perceived by mother, and this constitutes an evidence of excellent fetal state. If one is not careful, one may make the major mistake of taking the upper FHR tracing (hump level) as the baseline tachycardia (160 bpm) and diagnose the lower FHR tracing (120–130 bpm) as episodes of deceleration and take a wrong decision.

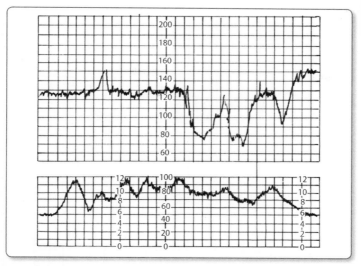

Fig. 13.17 FHR response to hyperstimulation of uterus

Deceleration with Fetal Movement (Fig. 13.19)

This antenatal CTG tracing shows deceleration with fetal movement rather than acceleration which is not a good sign. Please also note compensatory tachycardia which should not be mistaken for simple acceleration. Though there is no abnormality in baseline FHR the baseline variability is flatened. This was a case of IUGR at thirty eight weeks with diminished liquor and maternal complaint of diminished fetal movement. There occurred no contraction during the monitoring session of twenty minutes. Such cases may have further assessment by conducting ultrasonographic biophysical scoring specially estimation of the amniotic fluid index. Repeat CTG with or without acoustic stimulation also may be done. In all such cases, for taking decision, the other clinical parameters and inducability of the case also need to be assessed. This patient had LSCS on the same day and Apgar was eight. Liquor was scanty and it was heavily meconium stained.

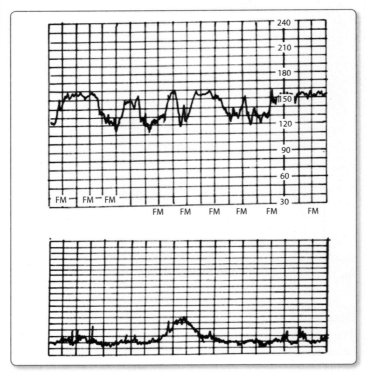

Fig. 13.18 Active awake fetus

Variable Deceleration (Fig. 13.20)

This multigravida who was admitted in advanced labor was found to have very irregular FHS on ordinary auscultation. So, she was put on CTG which showed this profound variable deceleration typical of cord compression though the cord was not felt on vaginal examination. Unfortunately, since the important basic parameter of frequency of contraction has not been traced here 'the element of variability' of deceleration in relation to contraction (see Chapter 12—CTG Interpretation—Theoretical Considerations') cannot be clearly established

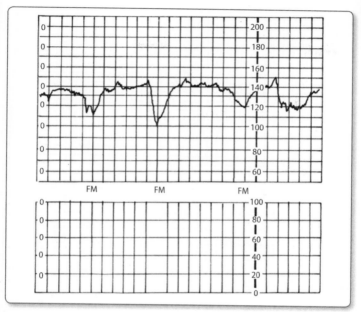

Fig. 13.19 Deceleration with fetal movement

on this tracing. Anyway, she was taken up for cesarean section but delivered normally in the operation theatre one hour and five minutes later. At delivery the cord was found to be significantly short and was tightly wound round the baby's neck. Though the baby come out with Apgar ten at one minute, had the delivery been delayed, it would certainly have developed severe hypoxia and acidosis.

Variable Deceleration (Fig. 13.21)

This is another tracing of variable deceleration with cord prolapse. The tracing shows a series of typical, three phased, 'M' shaped pattern each constituted by two episodes of acceleration, corresponding to the two upgoing apices of the letter 'M' with one episode of

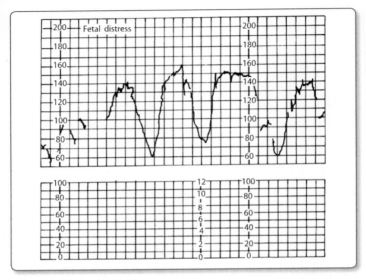

Fig. 13.20 Variable deceleration

deceleration in the middle—corresponding to the middle dipped portion of the letter 'M'.

Steer (1986) explained that the initial acceleration before deceleration occurs as a result of a compensatory phenomenon occasioned by 'partial compression' of the cord, i.e. when only venous flow through the cord is obstructed leading to decreased venous return to the fetal heart. On the phase of this deficiency the heart compensates by increasing its rate. The phase of deceleration which immediately follows the initial acceleration is attributed to reflex stimulation of vagal centre due to activation of aortic stretch receptors as a result of further compression of the cord now causing obstruction even to the arterial blood flow through cord (as the blood can no longer come to the placenta from fetus it accumulates in its aorta and causes the stretch). The phase of tachycardia which follows the deceleration phase is reactive and compensatory in nature

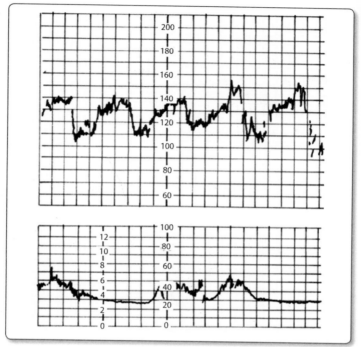

Fig. 13.21 Variable deceleration

and occurs as the compression on cord is released. This baby was delivered by emergency cesarean section and the Apgar was only three at one minute.

Variable Deceleration-Follow Up (Fig. 13.22)

Note an isolated but typical variable deceleration at the beginning of the FHR recording of this tracing which is of the so called 'M' shape. There is acceleration at the beginning and at the end of deceleration (with a dip in between). It is to be called variable because it has not come with every contraction, it has come with only one contraction out of three

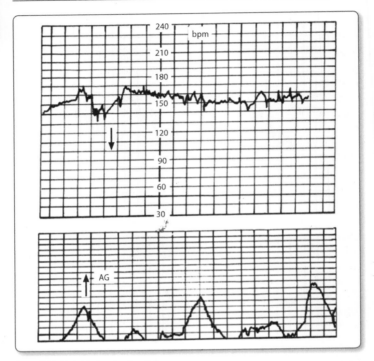

Fig. 13.22 Variable deceleration-follow up

during the ten minutes of tracing that is depicted here. Deceleration is of mild degree. FHR dropped only upto 140 bpm. There is good baseline variability even during deceleration phase. The only worrying thing in this tracing is that there is post-deceleration baseline tachycardia (not mere transient acceleration) lasting for nearly three minutes. Baseline FHR here varied between 150 and 160 bpm. This trace can also be classed as an *isolated type II deceleration* because there is typical time lag between the peak of contraction and nadir of deceleration.

This tracing was from a twenty seven years old normotensive primi at thirty nine plus weeks who came with leaking of clear liquor and was on oxytocin drip. As she kept having only occasional variable deceleration with normal tracing in between she was allowed to progress with hourly CTG and clinical monitoring in between. When she was put on CTG for the third time the deceleration was found to occur more frequently and it was sometimes synchronous and sometimes asynchronous with contraction. In view of this an emergency cesarean section was done. Vaginal examination in OT just prior to cesarean revealed cord prolapse. The baby was narrowly saved.

Variable Deceleration (Fig. 13.23)

The 'M' shaped pattern is very obvious in this tracing. Two noteworthy points here are—firstly, there is almost total loss of baseline variability (no saw-teeth), secondly, the deceleration had come in very quick succession allowing almost no time for recovery of FHR—both of which are of very ominous significance. Note that baseline FHR is not always easy to spot in the tracings of variable deceleration and needs critical look. The baseline FHR in this case would appear to be rather low (between 110–120 bpm).

Variable Deceleration due to Head Compression in Second Stage of Labor (Fig. 13.24)

This 'M' shaped FH tracing is typical of variable deceleration (unfortunately toco tracing has not been done in this case to precisely prove the lack of definite relation of the dips with uterine contraction). Notice the high baseline, i.e. the baseline tachycardia of 170–175 bpm. Baseline variability is also quite flatened under 5. The dips are quite deep reaching the level of 90 bpm. The patient delivered normally within one hour while preparations were being made for cesarean section and the baby was not affected. Though occult cord prolapse was excluded by PV before delivery—the possibility of cord compression due to lack of liquor (she had been leaking for six days) could not be ruled out.

Sinusoidal Pattern (Fig. 13.25)

A FHR tracing is considered to show sinusoidal pattern when both the 'amplitude' and the 'period' of variation of FHR show more or less

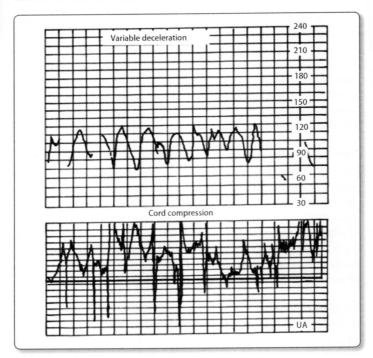

Fig. 13.23 Variable deceleration

constant value depicting a somewhat regular pattern. In this tracing the amplitude of variation was about 10 bpm and the period (i.e. the interval between variations) was about twenty seconds. Sinusoidal pattern with an amplitude of more than 25 bpm is considered ominous. Also notice in the tracing—a small degree of baseline tachycardia upto about 160 bpm.

This tracing was taken from an uncompleted postdated case in early labor. Notice that contractions were rather frequent—one in every two minutes. This sinusoidal FHR pattern in this case made its appearance only intermittently with normal tracing in between.

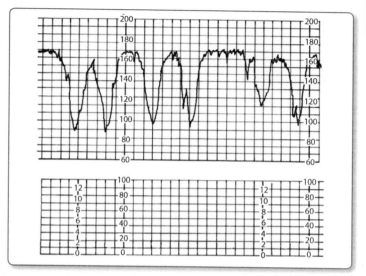

Fig. 13.24 Variable deceleration due to head compression in second stage of labor

The patient delivered normally after about six hours with Apgar nine and the baby was not anemic. Such cases of intermittent sinusoidal pattern with normal tracing in between can be considered as normal but calls for continuous monitoring.

Vibroacoustic Stimulation Test (VAST) (Fig. 13.26)

This was a case of mild pregnancy induced hypertension with mild IUGR at 38 weeks. While she was having her NST done—very poor baseline variability was noticed (see first part of the tracing) and so an acoustic stimulation was given. Note the instant response of the fetus by lot of movements and instant response of FH by sustained acceleration by over 20 bpm. It has to be appreciated that here the spikes in uterine contraction channel following the stimulation was caused by fetal movement and not by uterine contraction (paper speed—1 cm/min).

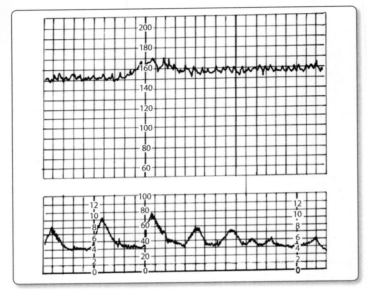

Fig. 13.25 Sinusoidal pattern

Tracing with poor baseline variability often needs 'prolonged' CTG monitoring to see whether it recovers or not, whether FM occurs or not, etc. Application of acoustic stimulation and judging the response it elicits often settles the matter within a very short time thereby saving time, expense and discomfort.

(Please read Chapter 19 – 'Vibroacoustic Stimulation Test (VAST) by CTG' before reading the analysis of next five tracings).

Vibroacoustic Stimulation Test (Fig. 13.27)

This is another tracing of fetal Vibroacoustic stimulation test in a case of uncomplicated postdated pregnancy with diminished fetal movement count (DFMC). As is evident in the tracing— stimulation showed a very reactive fetus with high (more than 180 bpm) acceleration and lot of fetal movement. Notice that at the

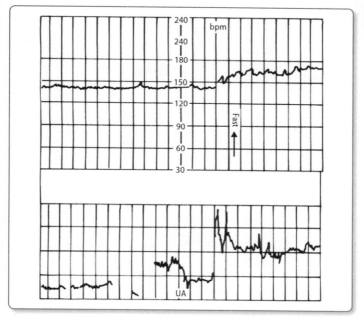

Fig. 13.26 Fetal Vibroacoustic stimulation test (VAST)

height of acceleration both short term and long term variability were almost completely lost. Looking at the tracing critically, though the VAST was reactive, the prolonged tachycardia (180–190) and also total loss of baseline variability it caused was somewhat non-reasuring.

This tracing was taken at paper speed of 2 cm/min. Compare this with the last tracing of VAST (**Fig. 13.26**) which was taken at 1 cm/minute and notice how the events are more spread out in this tracing in comparison to the last tracing.

Atypical Spiky VAST (Fig. 13.28)
Primi twenty one years, uncomplicated pregnancy at term + seven days with FM chart showing fourteen movements in three hours. In

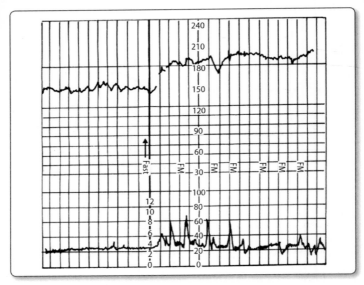

Fig. 13.27 Fetal Vibroacoustic stimulation test

view of postmaturity this CTG was done as a matter of routine for fetal monitoring. As poor baseline variability (2–5 bpm) was noticed in the tracing, Vibroacoustic stimulation was given. On first stimulus, although there occurred one FM and two accelerations by 15 bpm but both lasted for less than ten seconds producing a spiky shape. Not only this, there was also a spiky deceleration (see tracing). So, a second stimulus was given after two minutes. This induced one movement but again with spiky transient accelerations with tendency for FHR to drop below baseline rate on the return (The two stimuli are marked by two arrows on the tracings and the two FM by the letters FM). Monitoring was continued until the baseline variability returned to normal (5–10 bpm) which took about twenty-five minutes (description continued in the next, **Fig. 13.29**).

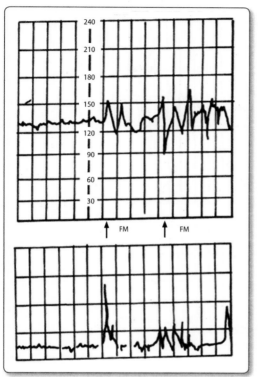

Fig. 13.28 Atypical spiky VAST

Atypical Spiky VAST (Fig. 13.29)

This is repeat CTG of the patient described in the last **Figure 13.28**—done one and half hours later. Notice, after three minutes of low variability an acoustic stimulation was given (marked by an arrow on the tracing) which caused one isolated barely qualifying acceleration, but soon after that variability again turned low. So, a second stimulus was given after two minutes (see second arrow) which caused spiky response just as in **Figure 13.28**, i.e. acceleration immediately followed by deceleration below baseline instead of sustained acceleration as

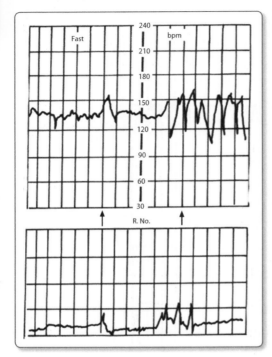

Fig. 13.29 Atypical spiky VAST

seen with healthy fetus (compare with **Figs 13.26** and **13.27**). The patient was induced immediately and on rupture of membranes thick meconium was found. So, she was taken up for cesarean section. The baby was born with Apgar two at one minute and five at five minutes, it weighed 2.3 kg. It was found to be grossly growth retarded which was missed antenatally.

An Unusual Response to VAST (Fig. 13.30)

Primi, thirty three years, at thirty eight week, IUGR by four weeks by Debdas' growth tape (ultrasound—not done), normotensive, spontaneous onset of labor. No bag, only few ml. of clear liquor came out on

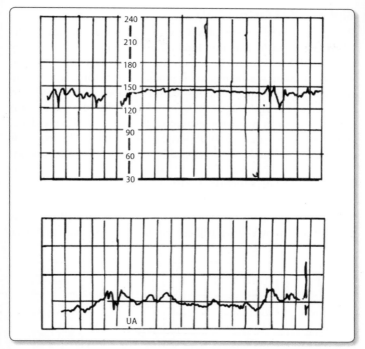

Fig. 13.30 An unusual response to VAST

doing ARM. The CTG was done as 'admission test'. FH in the first part of tracing shows normal baseline rate and normal baseline variability. But it became absolutely flat (straight line) immediately after giving a Vibroacousic stimulation. Though four movements were felt by the mother during this flat period but there was no acceleration with these. Note, after the second stimulus though variability improved a bit but it stayed around five only. After two hours a repeat 1 second VAST was given which showed multiple deceleration down to 70 bpm. An emergency cesarean was done. The Apgar was 10 but the baby was growth retarded and weighed only 2.08 kilogram.

Biphasic VAST (Fig. 13.31)

Primi, nineteen years, term plus two weeks, normotensive, induced by ARM and oxytocin drip, thin meconium in liquor. Trace shows very poor variability (almost like straight line) in the first half. A Vibroacoustic stimulus was then given. It produced first a large acceleration then a deceleration upto 90 bpm—followed by acceleration—followed by deceleration again upto 90 bpm. Notice, that the patient was contracting one in two to three minutes. Emergency LSCS was done. Apgar was 6 at 1 minute. Birth weight was 2.66 kg. The fetus, left alone perhaps would have developed more severe CTG abnormality.

Episodes of Deceleration (Fig. 13.32)

This tracing shows two sharp and deep dips in matter of fifteen minutes. This is an antenatal tracing which was done by external method. It was taken twenty minutes after artificial rupture of membranes to induce

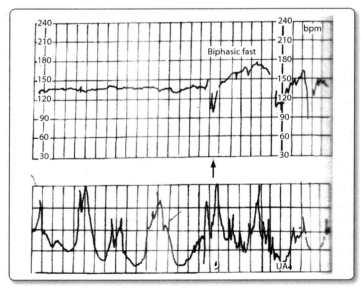

Fig. 13.31 Biphasic VAST

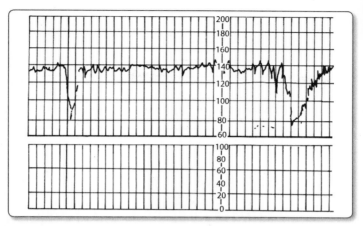

Fig. 13.32 Episodes of deceleration

labor. The liquor on amniotomy was thickly meconium stained. The patient was a primigravida aged thirty years at thirtyninth week and had been suffering from mild (130/90–140/90 mm of Hg) nonproteinuric pregnancy induced hypertension. Her fetus was clinically grossly growth retarded (7 weeks less by Debdas' growth tape) and she also had clinical oligohydramnios. Her FM count was borderline. As can be seen, apart from the dips, the baseline variability was also poor. However, in absence of simultaneous uterine contraction graph it is not possible to comment on the real significance of the dips. The dips could either be due to cord compression which is a probable association of oligohydramnios, and it is possible that drainage of some liquor following amniotomy had increased the likelihood of cord compression; but, all the same, these dips may well represent variable deceleration or late decelerations following two unrecorded uterine contraction. The patient had cesarean section soon after the tracing was taken. The baby weighed 1.2 kg and scored eight at one minute in Apgar's score.

Progressive Baseline Bradycardia (Fig. 13.33)

This young third gravida was post-dated by twenty one days and was induced by oxytocin drip and ARM. Her baseline FHR was

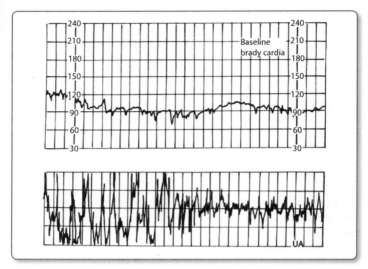

Fig. 13.33 Progressive baseline bradycardia

around 120 bpm with good variability at the time of induction. At ARM only a small amount of liquor came out and that was thickly meconium stained. Soon she developed sustained bradycardia down to 70–90 bpm also with poor variability. Uterine contraction tracing shows hyperstimulation. So, Syntocinon was stopped. An emergency cesarean was done. Baby weighed 2.7 kg and Apgar was seven at one minute.

Atypical Acceleration with Contraction (Fig. 13.34)

On first look it is difficult to ascertain which is the baseline FHR in this tracing whether the upper one which was running at 180 bpm or the lower one which was running between 110–120 bpm. On re-look it will be noticed that the upper tracing is precisely coinciding with the peak of every uterine contraction and lasting for a very short time. During the in-between contraction period, FHR can be seen to be

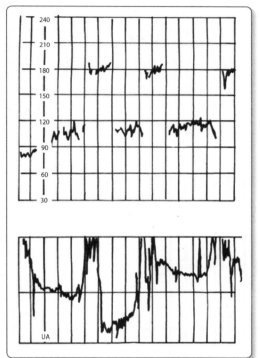

Fig. 13.34 Atypical acceleration with contraction

settling at its lower range which actually is the real baseline. Notice the baseline variability is well-preserved both during contraction and also in-between contraction. This uncomplicated case with mature fetus was kept under continuous monitoring and had a normal delivery after five hours with Apgar ten.

The explanation that has been put forward as the cause of such 'periodic acceleration' is—contraction stimulates fetal movement which in turn causes acceleration. However, it should be remembered that such a periodic 'big jump' in FHR may also be caused by momentary cord compression and hence such cases need continuous observation.

Uterine Polysystole (Fig. 13.35)

Examine the toco tracing first. Note that there occurred three contractions in a row without any relaxation but the patient was not very uncomfortable. This patient was induced by oxytocin infusion. Note the baseline tachycardia of almost 170 bpm. Notice one clear type I dip coinciding with the first peak of contraction, and a possible type II dip soon after that. All these disappeared as the oxytocin drip was omitted.

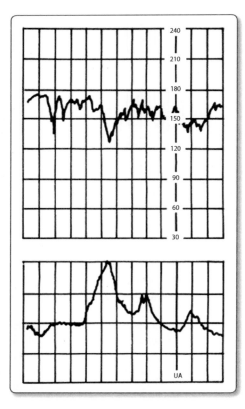

Fig. 13.35 Uterine polysystole

Admission Test (Fig. 13.36)

The principle of 'Admission test' is to assess *all* patients (not only high risk cases) cardiotocographically right on admission in labor in order to see how the fetus was behaving on the face of stress of intermittent constriction of its blood supply due to uterine contraction and on the basis of the findings of this test to plan the management of labor.

This booked young primigravida with uncomplicated pregnancy was admitted in early spontaneous labor at 38 weeks. On admission, a CTG was done as a part of 'Admission test' which showed a normal baseline FHR but poor baseline variability (1–3 bpm) and no accelera-

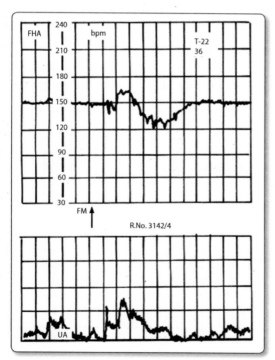

Fig. 13.36
Admission test

tion. However, no deceleration, spontaneous or contraction induced, was noticed over fifteen minutes period.

Instead of prolonging the monitoring, a Vibroacoustic stimulation was given which showed, as is evident in the tracing, a bi-phasic response, i.e. a prompt acceleration followed by a prolonged (of nearly two minutes duration) deceleration of about 30 bpm magnitude. Though mother recorded one movement immediately prior to application of stimulus, she felt no movement after the stimulus. After the deceleration, though FHR went back to its previous baseline rate but the same state of poor variability persisted. Artificial rupture of membranes was done immediately when scanty but clear liquor was drained. She was only 3 cm dilated. Since a repeat Vibroacoustic stimulation after thirty min. again showed poor response she was taken up for cesarean section. Baby weighed 2.3 kg and its Apgar was 5.

Scalp Stimulation Test (Fig. 13.37)

This patient in labor was having prolonged (over fifty minutes) low baseline variability. A PV was done to assess the progress of

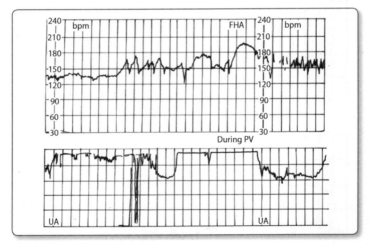

Fig. 13.37 Scalp stimulation test

labor and during PV FH showed marked acceleration through incidental plus intentional digital scalp stimulation. Not only this, the stimulation was followed by return of good baseline variability (see the last bit of the tracing). Such acceleration of FH through scalp stimulation is considered as a re-assuring sign of fetal well-being.

Scalp Stimulation Test (Fig. 13.38)

This primigravida with thin meconium in spontaneous labor at term had a PV at 4 cm dilatation when the fetus was given a digital scalp stimulation which showed instant significant acceleration of FH upto 15 bpm lasting for six minutes as shown in the tracing. The patient

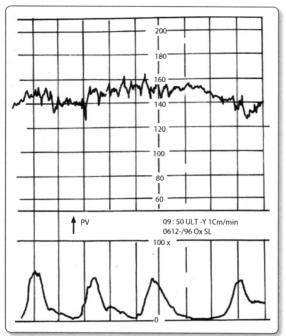

Fig. 13.38
Scalp
stimulation test

was kept under intermittent CTG monitoring and she delivered eight
hours later with 10 Apgar.

Scalp Stimulation Test (Fig. 13.39)

This tracing proposes to show the effect of digital overstimulation of
the fetal scalp. The onset of application of stimulus has been shown
by an arrow. As the stimulus was started there was acceleration of FH
by 20 bpm lasting for full sixty seconds which would lend the conclusion that the fetus was reactive. But notice soon after this acceleration
there was sudden deceleration by 30 bpm from the baseline. This
happened because at that point of time the pressure put on the scalp
was too high which acted like head compression (as in type I dip)
and caused this deceleration through vagal centre stimulation. As the
finger moved and the pressure eased there was again acceleration—
this time by 30 bpm from baseline and lasted for forty five seconds.
Again, next, as the finger pressure on the scalp was increased—again

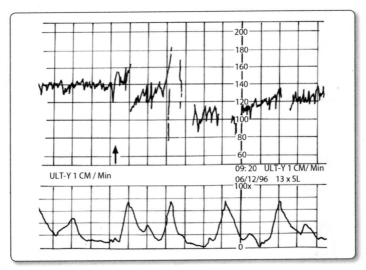

Fig. 13.39 Scalp stimulation test

there was deceleration—this time down to 90 bpm. However, notice that FH recovered soon after that as the pressure from the skull was eased and by the time vaginal examination was over FH returned to normal. The point to realise here is—one has to stimulate the scalp and not the skull or rather the skull content.

Effect of Pethidine on FHR Tracing (Fig. 13.40)

Notice the marked difference between first half and second half of the tracing, i.e. before and after the injection of Pethidine 100 mg and Phenargan 25 mg to the mother. The differences are as follows: marked reduction in the number and amplitude of FM acceleration, marked reduction in baseline variability and some reduction in baseline FHR after the injection in comparison to the state before the injection. Note that the mother recorded at least one movement before the injection but none after the injection. The point of time when the injection was given has been marked on the chart by an arrow.

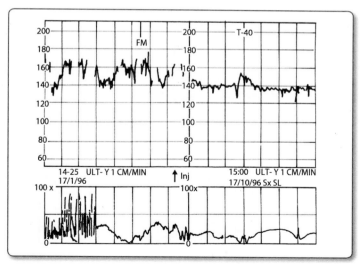

Fig. 13.40 Effect of pethidine on FHR tracing

Effect of Diazepam on FHR Tracing (Fig. 13.41)

This is an antenatal CTG (thirty six plus weeks) in a case of essential hypertension (on Labetalol 50 mg TDS) with superimposed pregnancy induced hypertension – showing the effect of IV Diazepam injection (10 mg) on FHR. Even previous to Diazepam injection CTG although had normal baseline (130 bpm) but was flat though reactive (not shown) – probably ? the effect of Labetalol. Within few seconds of the injection the baseline FHR dropped by 20 bpm and the baseline variability continued to be flat. As even ten minutes after the injection there was no sign of recovery of baseline and its variablity—an acoustic stimulation was given to which the fetus responded instantly by making some movement and by temporarily accelerating its heart by 20 bpm lasting for ninety seconds (paper speed—1 cm/minute). However, the drugged pattern of baseline bradycardia and reduced baseline variability soon returned. FH pattern returned to normal in all respects only after one hour twenty minutes.

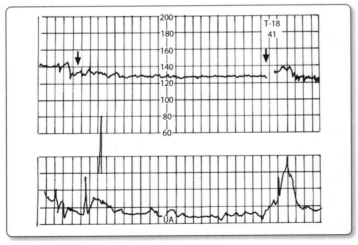

Fig. 13.41 Effect of Diazepam on FHR tracing

Iatrogenic CTG Abnormalities (Fig. 13.42)

This tracing was taken from a patient near term whose labor was induced for severe pregnancy induced hypertension. Note she is having rather frequent contractions (one in every two minutes) with little relaxation in between—a happening which was not recognisable clinically by palpation. The cause for this is hyperstimulation by oxytocin. Baseline FHR was within normal limits (though a bit on the lower side—122 bpm) but the baseline variability was grossly suppressed. This and also the somewhat lower baseline were Diazepam effect which the patient received (10 mg) a short while before. It is noteworthy that in this tracing both FH and uterine contraction abnormality were iatrogenic. Note total absence of FM,

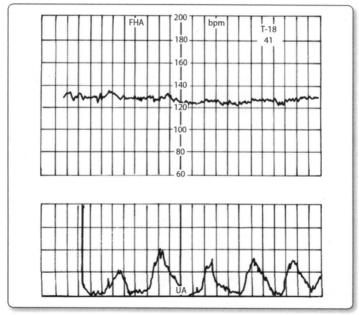

Fig. 13.42 Iatrogenic CTG abnormalities

FM acceleration, and even that of spontaneous acceleration of FH. The appropriate management in such a case would be—reduction in dose of oxytocin and assessment of FH response to Vibroacoustic stimulation (VAST) and, of course, continuous CTG monitoring until everything had returned to normal.

CTG Characteristics of Pre-term Pregnancy (Fig. 13.43)

This antenatal tracing was taken from an uncomplicated primigravida at thirty second week. The features characteristic of pre-term pregnancy in this tracing are: multiple spontaneous decelerations and total absence of acceleration even when actograph recorded fetal movement (note the thick dark line at the top part of the toco section of the CTG paper). Mother recorded four movements (Note the small dark vertical lines at the right upper corner of the tracing) and there was acceleration in this segment.

CTG Characteristics of Pre-Term Pregnancy (Fig. 13.44)

This uncomplicated primigravida was admitted with threatened premature labor at thirty three weeks of gestation. Notice the baseline tachycardia (170 bpm) and almost total absence of baseline variability both of which are known to be found in pre-term pregnancy even in absence of hypoxia. However, since these are very definite features of fetal compromise in the case of a mature fetus—such findings cause a lot of confusion and anxiety. In this case even at the end of three hours the same pattern persisted. Superimposition of late and/or variable deceleration on this pattern would, however, call for immediate interference. This tracing was taken before starting the tocolytic therapy. After nearly four hours of high anxiety, FH pattern became normal.

Mother's pulse and temperature were normal throughout.

Sequence of FHR Pattern from Fetal Distress to Fetal Death (Fig. 13.45)

This tracing alongwith the next tracing (**Fig. 13.46**), which is a continuity of this tracing after a short gap, constitutes a set of rare tracing

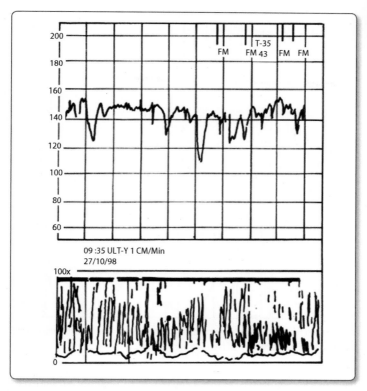

Fig. 13.43 CTG characteristics of pre-term pregnancy

which depict the sequence of events in FHR pattern—*from fetal distress to fetal death* in a case in labor. Notice the very first part of the tracing—it shows baseline tachycardia between 165–170 per minute and also poor baseline variability of 2–3 bpm. Immediately following this is noticeable three consecutive type II dips of the amplitude of 25 bpm and of the duration of two to 2 to 2½ minutes each (paper speed 1 cm per minute). Now notice the segments of FHR tracing in between dips. It is apparent that even during this period of uterine quiescence the

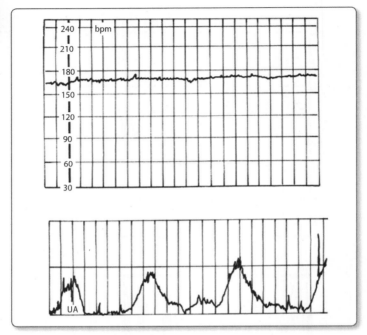

Fig. 13.44 CTG characteristics of pre-term pregnancy

baseline tachycardia has persisted and baseline variability continued to be poor. Notice the very end part of tracing and it will be observable that tachycardia here has mounted to 185 bpm.

Terminal FHR Pattern (Fig. 13.46)

As already mentioned, this is a continuity of **Figure 13.45**. It is quite obvious on the tracing that its first part is depicting severe bradycardia (a type II dip), its middle part showing an attempt towards compensation by pushing up the FHR and its last part showing profound terminal bradycardia with straight line FHR (almost total absence of baseline variability) until it all disappeared.

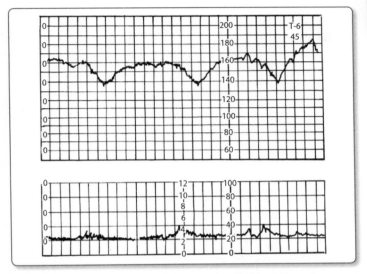

Fig. 13.45 Sequence of FHR pattern from fetal distress to fetal death. Notice three consecutive Type II dips, poor baseline variability and increasing tachycardia

This unbooked three days post-dated primigravida with BP of 140/100 was admitted with history of labor pain for about 12 hours. This fetus was growth retarded and liquor was thickly meconium stained. She was in second stage and had a low forceps delivery for benefit of doubt though FHS was absent and the baby was stillborn. It weighed 2.01 kilogram.

False Fetal Distress (Fig. 13.47)

This tracing is one of 'admission test'. Does not this tracing appear as an obvious example of very poor baseline variability of FH. Three acoustic stimulation also elicited no FH response (not shown in this tracing). Anyway, in view of this finding the tracing was continued while arrangements were being made for cesarean section.

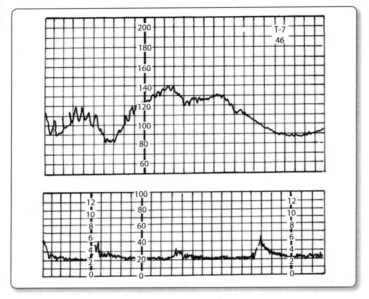

Fig. 13.46 Terminal FHR pattern

This unbooked third gravida, carrying near term pregnancy, who had one intrauterine death and one abortion in the past was admitted in early labor. One peculiar thing that was noticed in this case was although on tracing paper, FH was coming quite clearly with normal baseline rate (140/mm)—it could not be located by fetoscope at anytime. Checking of maternal pulse and maternal heart rate saved a cesarean section as the rate and rhythm of what appeared as FHS coincided with that of maternal pulse proving thereby that the signal was coming from maternal aorta and not from the heart of the fetus. The fetus in this case was already dead as confirmed later by ultrasound. This tracing emphasizes the importance of checking maternal pulse in every case. It also shows that it is a good practice to auscultate FH with fetoscope in every case at the beginning of CTG monitoring.

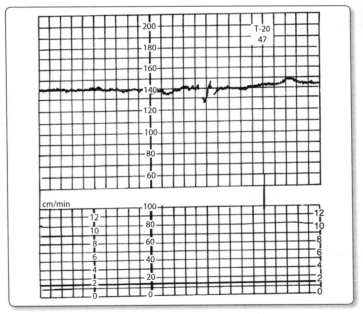

Fig. 13.47 False fetal distress

False Fetal Distress (Fig. 13.48)

This is a tracing from an unbooked primigravida at term with severe anemia and PIH. Though on admission FHS was absent on fetoscope examination, to confirm further the abdominal FH transducer was put on and this tracing, which is just like FH tracing, was obtained which caused a major confusion. So, to clear the confusion the transducer was put over maternal heart and similar sort of tracing was found to emerge. Mother's own pulse rate was 136 per minute. In such cases the US transducer happens to pick up maternal aortic pulsation. Intrauterine death was further confirmed by real time ultrasonography.

Ingemarsson et al (1993) reported similar false CTG tracing with dead fetus even when using direct fetal scalp electrode. It has

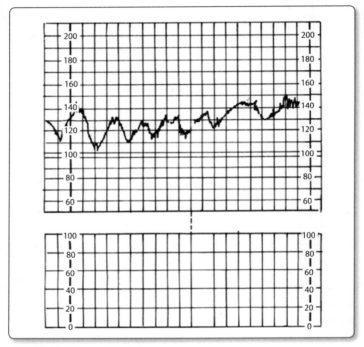

Fig. 13.48 False fetal distress

been suggested that, when the fetus is dead, the maternal 'R' wave are picked up by the scalp electrode as the next best signal and are counted by the Cardiotachometer (Cunningham et al, 2010) giving such confusing tracings.

Fetal Actocardiograph (Fig. 13.49)

This is a tracing of a false-positive antenatal NST as proved by actocardiograph. Notice in the first half of the tracing that there occurred three fetal movement (FM) as marked by three long pointed vertical lines at the top margin of the tracing towards the left which

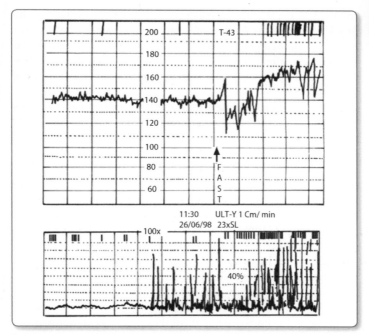

Fig. 13.49 Fetal actocardiograph

was registered by the mother through the remote event marker but no corresponding FHR acceleration occurred proving thereby that it was a non-reactive NST. Now notice that as on the 8th minute a Vibroacoustic stimulation was given there followed a surge of FM and instant acceleration of FHR to upto 170 bpm from the baseline of 140 proving thereby that it was a case of false-positive NST and here comes the role of actocardiography to objectively prove it as explained below.

Observe carefully the lower (toco) segment of the tracing. The tiny dark lines along its upper margin represent FM automatically recorded by the machine. Besides this, actocardiograph facility also provides another mechanism of depicting occurrence of FM which is in the form of a graph called 'actograph'. Note, in this particular tracing the graph facility was switched on only after the initial five minutes and notice that the actograph consists of multiple spikes of various heights.

Please also note that the actocardiograph machines also provides 'frequency filter threshold selector' facilty of the range between 0–99 percent which means one can choose upto what frequency of ultrasound returning from the various moving parts of the fetus one wants to use to activate the FM marker to record FM automatically by the machine and then printing the representative tiny dark lines at the top margin of toco segment of the tracing paper as described above. Notice the forty percent (40%) mark printed in the middle of actograph and hundred percent (100%) mark printed along the top line of toco segment of the paper. It has been found that with 40 percent filter the sensitivity of actogram is ninety six percent (96%) with mature fetus as double checked by simultaneous real-time ultrasound scan.

Notice in the tracing that after the Vibroacoustic stimulation when the fetus started making vigorous movements the frequency of ultrasound echoes generated by these movements crossed the 40 percent threshold level and automatically printed the series of tiny dark lines (see the last 4 minutes of the toco part of the tracing). As is evident from this tracing, the ease and objectivity of the actocardiograph is unparalleled specially for doing NST.

Biophysical Profile by Actocardiography (Fig. 13.50)

This tracing is from a patient with moderate IUGR who was extremely insensitive to her fetal movement. As is evident in the tracing, she could feel only one movement (see the top left corner of the tracing) during 14 minutes period shown here. Now see the small black acto marks printed along the top of toco channel. It is obvious from these marks that there have been a lot of movements and corresponding acceleration of FHR certifying that fetus is in good state. Now notice the 'frequency-

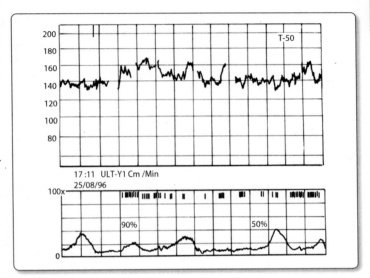

Fig. 13.50 Biophysical profile by actocardiography

filter' threshold marks. Some movements were so vigorous that it printed acto marks even with 90 percent filter. Notice, the filter threshold was reduced to 50 percent during later part of the tracing.

This movement profile and the corrosponding heart response along with intermittent amniotic fluid index (AFI) perhaps constitute the best biophysical profile of the fetus—the former depicting any acute hypoxic insult and the later the chronic compromise.

FURTHER READING

1. Arias E. Practical guide to high-risk pregnancy and delivery, 2nd edition, Mosby Year Book, St Louis, 1993;3–20, 301–18 and 413–29.
2. Arulkumarn S. Obstetrics and Gynaecology for postgraduates, 1st edition, edited by Ratnam SS, Bhaskar Rao, K and Arulkumaran S, Orient Longman, Madras, India, 1992;115–26.

3. Beard RW, Filshie GM, Knight CA, Roberts GM. J Obstet Gynaecol Br C With, 1971;78:865–81.

4. Cunningham FG, Leveno KJ, Bloom SL, et al, in William's Obstetrics, 23rd Edition, Intrapartum Assessment, Mc Graw Hill, New York, 2010;410–43.

5. Debdas AK. J Obst Gynae of India 1996;46:497–500.

6. Debdas AK. Practical Cardiotocography, Published by Fetal Monitoring Research Centre, Jamshedpur, 1993;56–74.

7. FIGO. "Guidelines for the use of fetal monitoring" Int J Obstet Gynecol 1993;25:159–67.

8. Fleischer A, Schulman H, Jagani N, Mitchell J, Randolph G. Am J Obstet Gynecol 1982;144:55–60.

9. Flynn AM, Kelly J. Recent Advances in Obst and Gynae, Edited By John Bonnar, Vol-14, Churchill Livingstone 1982;25–45.

10. Fraser DM and Cooper MA in Myles Textbook for Midwives, 15th Edition, Monitoring the Fetus, Churchill Livingstone, London, , 2009;481–4.

11. Ingemarsson I, Ingemersson E, Spencer JAD. Fetal heart rate monitoring a practical guide, Oxford University Press, Oxford, 1993;178–79, 283–85.

12. Magowan B, Owen P, Drife J: Clinical Obst Gynae, 2nd edition, Monitoring the Fetus in labor, Elsevier, Edinburg, 2009;331–43

13. Mishell DR, Kirschbaum TH, Morrow CP. Year Book of Obstetrics and Gynaecology-1993. Edited by these authors, Year book publisher, Chicago, 1993;136–62.

14. NICE (National Institute for Clinical Excellance) Guideline :The use of Electronic fetal monitoring: the use and interpretation of Cardiotocography in Intrapartum Fetal Surveillance, London, 2001

15. NICE (National Institute for Clinical Excellance) Guideline :The Clinical Guideline No. 70, Induction of labour, RCOG press, London, 2008

16. Steer PJ. Fetal heart rate patterns and their clinical interpretations, Oxford Sonicaid Ltd, Sussex, UK, 1986;1–44.

Problems in Interpretation of CTG and Solution

This problem is a bit more clinically serious for antenatal CTG monitoring than for intranatal CTG monitoring because the former entails the additional risk of induced premature delivery of the fetus if the findings get labelled 'falsely' unsatisfactory, i.e. in the case of a false positive result. However, on the contrary, it is noteworthy that the procedure of *antenatal CTG is more amenable to standardisation* than CTG in labor because of the following reasons:

a. In the case of antenatal monitoring the duration of monitoring can be standardised and fixed (say at 15 or 20 minutes) which may not be a very logical course for a dynamic event like labor specially because the goings here may be further modified by the variable factors like variable amplitude and frequency of uterine contraction. Actually, **standardisation of duration of monitoring** is a very necessary element for ensuring uniform interpretation because, for example, if one unit fixes the duration of monitoring at 15 minutes and the other at 45 minutes, it is quite possible for the result of interpretation to vary, for, with longer monitoring, some transient abnormalities may disappear where as, in some instances, some new abnormality may appear.

b. Antenatal CTG is also free of such modifying external factors as the effect of variable types and doses of sedatives and analgesics— the use of which is almost universal for cases in labor.

THE NATURE OF PROBLEM

Though CTG has become an integral part of obstetric practice over the last 45 years, specially in the developed countries, yet criticism about the difficulty in its interpretation still continues. A study in this regard was conducted by Kieth et al (1995) who asked each of 17 experts to review 50 tracings on two occasions at least one month apart and found that 20 per cent changed their own interpretation and 25 per cent did not agree with the interpretation of their colleagues. Apparently the problem seems to be:

a. Lack of clarity of definition of both normal and abnormal CTG.
b. Lack of uniformity about the number of criteria to be evaluated for labelling abnormal from normal.
c. Lack of agreement about the importance to be given to each criteria, and
d. The dependence on visual analysis.

These lead to the following clinical problems:

1. High false positivity rate—which means abnormal CTG report but normal fetal pH and normal Apgar.
2. High rate of intervention specially induction and cesarean section.
3. Occasional fetal demise or birth of brain-damaged baby for not giving enough gravity to certain set of CTG finding.

In contrast to above, Ayres-de-Campose et al (1999) reported—"Trained observers will agree on abnormal and normal fetal heart rate traces, however defined, on 83 occasions out of 100; and will agree on the question of intervention, however defined, on 87 occasions out of 100".

Endeavour Towards Solution
Clinical

- CTG scoring system.
- CTG color coding

Gadgetry

- Automatic computer analysis of the tracing and online reporting.

    (See Chapter 20—"Computer Analysis of CTG Trace"—an exclusive chapter devoted on this method).

    Note: This method is however applicable for antenatal CTG monitoring only.

CTG SCORING SYSTEM

In order to increase reliability and to bring in ease and uniformity many researchers over the last 3 decades have tried to formulate scores. Given below are the criteria on which the scoring systems have generally been based:

- Baseline FHR.
- FHR response to FM.
- FHR response to uterine contraction.
- Amplitude of beat-to-beat variation, and
- Frequency of such variation.

    Depending on the degree and frequency at which a particular criterion presents itself, it is given the score 0, 1, 2 just as in Apgar's score.

    Though it sounds very logical, scientific, and easy yet in practice it has been found to be far from it as has been detailed below.

Problems with the Scoring System

1. No uniformity in the number of criteria to be evaluated, e.g. some authors take three criteria and evaluate on $3 \times 2 = 6$ total points while some authors take five criteria and evaluate on $5 \times 2 = 10$ total points.
2. No uniformity in the degree of importance to be attached to a criterion.
3. Some criteria are difficult to assess and capture in numerical definition (i.e. quantify), e.g. short-term fluctuations.

4. Some criteria need tracing for a long time which is expensive and time consuming and also tiring and worrisome for the patient. For example, it is difficult to find the relationship of FHR with contraction in NST because Braxton-Hicks contraction may not come for a long time.

5. The 50 per cent score, which is often taken as the cutoff point, can be achieved by too many combinations, e.g. for Pearson and Weaver's 'six point score' by seven combinations and Meyer Menk's 'ten point' score by 51 combinations (Pearson, 1981).

6. Being a bit cumbersome, whereas not very obviously beneficial, the conformity of obstetric staff to score every CTG has been found to be very low.

As can be seen from the above review that trying to score CTG is not the right avenue to solve the CTG interpretation problem. Hence, in the recent years, obstetric scientists are concentrating in developing a 'double check system' to re-confirm the non-reassuring traces.

COLOR CODING OF CTG TRACES

Parer and Ikeda (2007) identified 134 patterns of intrapartum tracing and color coded each pattern using green and red color. Those falls in the green code do not need any action and those fall in red code need prompt delivery. But no joy. Complexity remained.

FURTHER READING

1. Ayres-de-Campose, et al. Grant JM (Ed). Editor's choice. Brit J Obstet Gynaecol 1999;vii:1307–10.

2. Debdas AK : Management of Non-reassuring Cardiographic (CTG) tracing; Practical Obstetrics, Jaypee Medical Publishers, New Delhi, 2003;147–50.

3. Keith RDF, Backley S, Garibaldi GM, et al. Brit J Obstet Gynaecol 1995;102:688.
4. Parer JTand Ikeda T: A framework for standardized management of intrapartum heart rate pattern: Am J Obstet Gynecol, 197:26 (2007)
5. Pearson JF. Progress in Obstetrics and Gynaecology. In: John Studd (Ed). Churchill Livingstone. 1981;1:105-24.

CHAPTER 15

Applied Cardiotocography— Antenatal

This chapter covers the following tests that can be done through the use of CTG to assess and predict antenatal fetal health:

I. Non-stress test (NST)
II. Contraction stress test (CST)
   • Oxytocin challenge test (OCT)
   • Nipple stimulation stress test (NSST)
III. Vibroacoustic stimulation test (VAST)—see Chapter 19
IV. Fetal actogram/actocardiogram
V. CTG assistance in daily fetal movement count (DFMC) by mother.

Problems of Monitoring Fetus during Antenatal Period

Monitoring fetus during antenatal period has always been a problem due to:

a. the physical inaccessibility of fetus
b. the silent nature of its diseases and distress—a matter which is worsened by the
c. unmanageably long length of time it needs to be monitored – at least three long months—the last trimester of pregnancy.

Biochemical tests which endeavoured to assess fetal state indirectly through assessment of placental function has now gone totally out of favor because of its poor predictability. Antenatal fetal monitoring for the last 40 years or so has been almost completely taken over by electronic fetal monitoring by cardiotocography which assesses a very vital, dynamic *'direct fetal parametre'*—the behavior of fetal heart, complemented by realtime ultrasonography giving fetal biophysical profile and liquor volume, and further refined by Doppler velocimetry in selected cases.

Specific Expectation from Antenatal CTG

As opposed to intranatal CTG monitoring where the emphasis is *on the present,* i.e. 'on the spot state' of fetus—the emphasis in antenatal fetal monitoring is on its *"predictive value"* for the continued satisfactory state of the fetus over, at least, next 48 hours—if not one week.

Each of the tests enumerated above has been detailed below one by one.

NON-STRESS TEST (NST)

This quick, easily interpreted (even by midwives and junior doctors) test was originally introduced as a 'screening test' of fetal well-being for antenatal population at large. The test aims to assess just one simple parameter that is—whether the FHR accelerates with the occurrence of fetal movement (FM) or not—*FM as sensed and registered by the mother.* The 'qualifying acceleration' for the purpose is—a minimum of 15 bpm rise of a minimum 15 seconds duration.

The results of the test is expressed simply as:

Reactive   –   If qualifying acceleration (15/15) has occurred at least 3 times in 20 minutes of observation period.

Non-reactive –   Non-occurrence of acceleration of the above description during the specified observation period.

The above single parameter test is, however, now considered incomplete and not very reliable since it does not take into account many other important FH parameter (as described below) and is associated with high false positivity rate. The original NST has now been enriched by adding five other important parametres to get a more reliable result out of it. Though after this quality parameter change, the procedure should be logically termed 'non-stress assessment' (NSA) rather than NST, but conventionally the old term NST is used synonymously for NSA also.

The Criteria to be Assessed in an NST/NSA Tracing

a. Baseline FHR
b. Baseline variability of FHR
c. FM acceleration—"the Key element"
d. Any-other acceleration
e. Any deceleration, if present, it's type
f. Any contraction, if present, it's frequency, duration, relation to FH behavior (amplitude of contraction is applicable only for internal monitoring which is possible only in labor after rupture of membranes).

What does the Word "Non-Stress" Imply?

The word 'non-stress' implies absence of stress of uterine contraction on fetus which, as is well known, intermittently threats the fetus by constricting the retroplacental blood vessels as in labor. The term non-stress is also used to differentiate this test (NST) from another antenatal cardiotocographic test called contraction stress tests (see below) where the stress for the fetus is generated artificially to assess the fetal response on the face of it.

Physiological Basis of Key Element of NST (i.e. FM Acceleration)

Occurrence of acceleration of FHR in response to FM indicates the occurrence of the following underlying physiological activity for which adequate fetal cerebral oxygenation is necessary:

a. Intact and responsive fetal central nervous system
b. Normal functioning of the mechanism of the reflex that brings on the cardiac adaptability to the above CNS activity.

Hence, in otherwise normal fetus whose mother has not received any CNS depressant drug—the non-occurence of FM acceleration can be taken as an evidence of inadequate oxygenation provided fetal sleep has been excluded.

Technique of doing NST

The patient is laid on bed in 15° left lateral tilt in order to minimise aortocaval compression. The FH transducer is belted on lower abdomen at a site from where the FH is most clearly audible and the toco transducer is belted on the upper abdomen over the uterine fundus so that it can easily detect the anterior deflection of uterus that occurs during a contraction. The 'patient button', which is actually a remote event marker, is given to the paitent so that she can press it as and when she feels any FM and as she does so a mark is printed on the CTG paper. This is a very necessary part of the procedure because by this only the FH acceleration can be precisely correlated with FM. Machine with actocardiography facility (see later in this chapter) also *automatically* senses and prints the occurrence of FM. Besides, the occurrence of FM can also sometimes be further confirmed by the sound it occasionally causes in the audio channel or a spike it may produce in toco channel.

Duration of Monitoring

The CTG machine should be run on –
- For a period of 20 minutes at the paper speed of 1 cm/min or
- Until three accelerations of at least 15 BPM lasting for at least 15 seconds have occurred (see above).

If such acceleration, which constitutes a reactive test, fails to occur within twenty minutes the machine should be run on for *another 20 minutes* to exclude the possibility that the test was being (incidentally) performed during the fetal sleep period (see Chapter 18 'Fetal Sleep, Rest, Activity and CTG').

Special allowance for Gross IUGR Cases

In such cases, some units continue the monitoring *until three Braxton-Hicks* contractions have occurred accepting the drawbacks such as—entails long period of monitoring, long engagement of man-time and machine-time (which may not always be practical), higher expense and discomfort for the patient. However, such investment may be worthwhile because occurrence of silent shallow late deceleration with Braxton-Hicks sometimes occur in some of these cases and may be decisive.

In the recent years, introduction of VAST (see Chapter 19) has made a major difference in the duration and objectivity of NST.

Interpretation of NST

This has already been described in details in Chapter12,13 and 14.

Here is to summarise:

CTG Interpretation Ready Reckoner

CTG characteristics of a well oxygenated fetus

1. Baseline FHR between 120 and 160 bpm.
2. Baseline variability > 5 bpm (5–15 bpm).
3. Minimum of two episodes of qualifying FH acceleration coincident with FM during the twenty minutes of tracing period.
4. Total absence of deceleration of any form.
5. Presence of qualifying acceleration even without FM. (Beard, 1974, Steer, 1986; Debdas, 1994).

    Besides the pattern described above, all other tracing pattern should be viewed with some suspicion (i.e. labelled as 'Non-reassuring') and be further evaluated.

CTG characteristics of a possibly compromised fetus

1. FHR above 160 bpm (tachycardia)
2. FHR below 110 bpm (bradycardia)
3. Baseline variability of < 5 bpm
4. Absence of qualifying acceleration with FM
5. Total absence of acceleration
6. Occurrence of 'Late deceleration' (see later) with Braxton-Hicks contraction. This is an early and a very reliable sign of fetal compromise.

7. Occurrence of any type of deceleration specially if it is of the magnitude of more than 15 bpm and lasting for more than 15 seconds (qualifying deceleration).
8. Total absence of FM.

Predictability of NST

False-negative Rate

This means reactive NST in a fetus who is actually in distress. Its incidence has been reported as—3 per 1000. So, it would appear that the likelihood of fetal death or its serious morbidity following a negative NST is extremely low (Arias, 1993).

False-positive Rate

This means non-reactive NST in a healthy fetus. Its incidence is very high—50 percent if only morbidity (e.g. low Apgar) is taken into account and 80 percent if mortality is taken into account (Arias, 1993).

Frequency of Antenatal CTG Testing

A good CTG tracing in otherwise normal patient is highly predictive of absence of fetal death within next seven days (Debdas, 1995; Cunningham et al, 1993). But for high-risk cases twice weekly testing is recommended. Many obstetricians perform daily or even more frequent CTG for certain very high-risk cases (Cunningham et al, 1993) and also for otherwise permium fetuses like for the fetuses of IVF pregnancy. It has been found that in antenatal cases, predictability of NST is better in chronic situations like in postdated pregnancy, pregnancy induced hypertension, IUGR, etc.

It needs to be emphasised that CTG surveillance **must be supplemented by** daily fetal movement count (**DFMC**) by mother in the in-between period.

In the cases that are proved to have diminished liquor, e.g. IUGR cases, postdated pregnancies, etc. CTG monitoring must be supplemented by intermittent amniotic fluid index (**AFI**) assessment by ultrasonography.

Where telemetry facility is available, CTG can be done at patient's house and the data can be transmitted to hospital through telephone link (Cunningham et al, 1993). This saves the patient from getting admitted to hospital and/or from taking the trouble of coming to hospital frequently for monitoring.

'Practical Policy' of Antenatal Fetal Monitoring by CTG

The CTG is not meant for monitoring the whole antenatal population. This is not only because the venture is impractical considering the unmanageable length of time to be monitored (a minimum of three months period) and unmanageable expense to be incurred but also for the fact that it will not be cost effective, for, this way, proportionately, only very few will be found abnormal for the enormous volume to be screened. Hence, for practical purpose, to derive the best benefit from antenatal CTG, it should be used in the following policy:

CTG as 'Dominant Method' of Fetal Monitoring

Only high-risk cases will come under this category like IUGR, post-dated pregnancy, cases with bad obstetric history, persistent PIH, APH, diabetics, etc.

CTG as a 'Secondary Method' of Fetal Monitoring

Under this indication comes are the cases where CTG is to be used just as 'fall back on' method and this includes the masses of low-risk or no-risk cases. In this clinically 'normal' cases the primary method of screening should be the daily fetal movement count (DFMC) and CTG should be used only in the cases showing low FM count.

Main Use of CTG for Antenatal Fetal Monitoring

Main use of antepartum CTG monitoring is to allow "more" women with "high-risk pregnancy" to continue their pregnancy–

- To greater maturity
- To safer maturity
- To better inducibility
  or

- Until the spontaneous onset of labor (widely quoted logical use).

Causes 'Other than Hypoxia' that can produce Abnormal CTG Tracing during Antenatal Period

1. *Pre-term fetus* Due to immaturity of their para-sympathetic system they may manifest some degree tachycardia and poor baseline variability.

2. *Post-term fetus* Rate between 100 and 120 can be considered as normal in post-term fetus provided all the other CTG parameters like baseline variability, FM acceleration, etc. are absolutely normal and there are no other clinical abnormality. (Steer, 1986).

3. *Maternal medication* Beta adrenergic drugs like ritodrine, balbutamol, etc. used to arrest premature labor may cause fetal tachycardia. On the other hand, atropine can cause the same by its parasympatholytic action. Narcotics (sedatives), barbiturates, phenothiazines (e.g. promethazine), tranquilizers (e.g. diazepam, librium), anticonvulsant (e.g. magnesium sulphate), metoclopramide, pethidine, morphine, etc. all can cause diminished baseline variability, i.e. flat CTG (Steer, 1986; Cunningham et al, 2010).

4. *Stress* Adrenaline and nonadrenaline released by mother and fetus in response to stressful stimuli have a powerful effect on FHR causing tachycardia (Steer, 1986).

5. *Supine hypotension* This can be associated with diminished baseline variability correctable on turning the patient to one side.

6. *Maternal pyrexia* Fever from any source can cause fetal tachycardia (Cunningham et al, 1993, 2010). Though the cause and effect relationship here is obvious, yet recurrent finding of such high tachycardia can be quite distressing for the Obstetrician. Besides, there remains the possibility of persistent tachycardia leading ultimately to heart failure.

7. *Severe maternal and fetal anemias* These may result in baseline tachycardia (Flynn and Kelly, 1982)—the glaring example of fetal anemia being severe hemolytic disease.

8. *Maternal cardiac failure* This also can produce fetal tachycardia (Flynn and Kelly, 1982).
9. *Fetal central nervous system abnormality* This may be associated with poor baseline variability.
10. *Fetal sleep*—see Chapter 18—"Fetal Sleep, Rest, Activity and CTG".
11. *Fetal cardiac abnormality* Fetal congenital heart block and cardiac arrhythmias can cause abnormal CTG tracing (Cunningham et al, 2010).

Planning Action on CTG Findings

Apart from the actual character of the tracing itself, the following factors must be given due consideration for planning action on CTG findings–

1. Whether any cause other than hypoxia that can produce FH changes and abnormal tracing are present or not (see above).
2. The total clinical situation of the case.
3. Gestational age/maturity of the fetus.
4. Volume of liquor present—specially whether AFI is low, i.e. less than five.
5. Color of liquor—for patients in labor with ruptured membranes.
6. Whether mother is on any medication that matters (see above).

Summary of Interrelation between Hypoxia and CTG Changes

1. *Baseline tachycardia* This occurs in cases of gradually developing hypoxia. It's purpose is to maintain oxygenation to vital centres by increasing the cardiac output. As fetal system is less able to increase its stroke volume, its heart rate has to go up to meet the increased demand (Arulkumaran, 1992).
2. *Baseline bradycardia*
   a. Fall of PO_2 in fetal blood (hypoxemia) stimulates chemo-receptors present in the carotid and aortic bodies and causes baseline bradycardia.

   b. Severe and more prolonged hypoxemia leads to tissue hypoxia—which in turn leads to metabolic acidosis. The latter causes more severe and prolonged baseline bradycardia through its direct effect on fetal myocardium (Cunningham et al, 1993, 2010).

3. *Reduction in baseline variability*
   a. Parasympathetic would appear to be mainly responsible for baseline variability and since in conditions of chronic hypoxia the para-sympathetic control is lost first, decreased variability results. Acute hypoxia, on the other hand, has been found to increase the variability (Cunningham et al, 1993) initially.
   b. In the severe and prolonged hypoxic situation culminating in metabolic acidosis, the reduced variability is brought about by the depression of fetal brainstem by acidaemia. In view of this, flat CTG is also considered a reflection of fetal acidemia rather than of just hypoxia. (Cunningham et al, 1993).

4. *Late deceleration* Steer (1986) has shown that late decelerations make their appearance only when the PO_2 of fetus falls below 10 mm of Hg and it is mediated through the chemoreceptors present in aortic and carotid body.

5. *Accelerations* If FHR pattern shows spontaneous qualifying accelerations the chance of the fetus developing acidosis is nil. As a corollary to this, absence of acceleration in any trace is generally recognised as one of the earliest features of hypoxia (Arulkumaran, 1992).

CONTRACTION STRESS TEST (CST)

This test, which is really a test for placental reserve, proposes to stress the fetus by partially obliterating the retroplacental blood vessels which feed the intervillous circulation—by artificially bringing about uterine contraction. A positive CST is considered as one of the earliest sign of fetal hypoxia (Arias, 1993).

Depending on how the contraction is brought about, CST can be classified into two types as follows:

- Oxytocin challenge test (OCT)
- Nipple stimulation stress test (NSST).

However, these are not practiced nowadays for reasons narrated below.

Oxytocin Challenge Test (OCT)

Method

It is exactly same as NST (see NST). After fixing the FH and toco discs on patient's abdomen the machine should be run on for 20 minutes for baseline observation.

Following this the patient is intravenously infused with increasing dosage of oxytocin with the help of slow injection pump until a contraction is stimulated. Oxytocin is started usually at 0.5 μ/min and increased (usually doubled) at interval of 15–20 minutes depending on the response until qualifying contraction is obtained (see below).

Since this test takes long time, one must make sure that the patient is not laid supine and kept slightly proped up and turned to her left side with the help of cushion in order to avoid vena caval compression. Patient's blood pressure should be taken every 10 minutes throughout.

After completion of the test, CTG monitoring should be continued for another 20–30 minutes to observe any residual effect or after-effect and until all contractions have died down.

In some cases it may be necessary to quieten the uterus by subcutaneous administration of 250 mg of terbutaline.

Qualifying Contraction

For a proper test—a minimum of three contractions, each lasting for 40 to 60 seconds, must occur within 10 minutes period (Arias, 1993).

Observation and Inference

- Occurrence of late deceleration with qualifying contraction constitutes *positive test*.
- Non-occurrence of late deceleration with qualifying contraction constitutes *negative test*. (Freeman, 1982).

- Occurrence of FH acceleration with contraction indicate existence of good placental reserve and well oxygenated fetus.

  If qualifying contraction fails to occur inspite of oxytocin dose of 16 µ/minute over a period of 1 1/2 to 2 hours—it is considered as test failure.

Indications of CST

Since the CST is somewhat invasive in nature it is generally used as a secondary test of fetal well-being, i.e. when the non-invasive tests like NST and biophysical profile (BPP) scoring show abnormal result. The idea is to double-check the state of the fetus with a superior test. This is expected to effect reduction of false positivity rate of the above two tests and thereby reduce the interference rate.

Predictability of CST

False negative rate—0.4 per 1000 (as opposed to 3.2/1000 for NST)
False positive rate—as high as *50 percent for fetal morbidity* (i.e. similar to NST) (Arias, 1993).

Nipple Stimulation Stress Test (NSST)

In this test also, with the patient in semi-fowler or slightly lateral position, baseline CTG is done for 15 to 20 minutes. Then a warm moist gauge piece or handkerchief is placed on one of the breasts of the patient and she is instructed to massage or roll her (that) nipple for 10 minutes while toco channel of CTG is continuously observed for occurrence of any contraction. If this has failed to produce any contraction she then massages both her nipples for a period of another ten minutes. Once the contraction begins—the stimulation is immediately stopped. Like OCT, aim here also is to elicit 3 contractions in ten minutes (see qualifying contraction).

Special Advantage of Contraction Stress Tests (CST) (i.e. OCT and NSST)

Since the qualifying criterion in both the contraction stress tests is the occurrence of late deceleration—a sign which has been shown both clinically and experimentally to be the earliest indicator of fetal compromise—these tests are considered as a more reliable test of fetal well-being than NST and BPP.

Drawbacks of CST

1. It is invasive specially OCT.
2. It has too many "contraindications like—APH, scarred uterus, patients with high-risk of going into premature labor, cases of premature rupture of membranes, incompetent cervix, multiple pregnancy, cases with known uterine malformation, etc.
3. It takes 1 1/2 to 2 hours to perform.
4. It needs close skilled supervision.
5. The test has poor patient acceptance—both OCT and NSST.
6. By causing uterine hypertonus it may constitute an iatrogenic hazard to the already compromised fetus. In this connection, Debdas and Kaur (1986) from their study of nipple stimulation stress test in 20 high-risk cases found as high as 45 percent meconium staining incidence rate in this group in comparison to a figure of only 18 percent amongst matched control group of high-risk cases who were followed with conventional unstressed CTG. Hill et al (1984) also reported nearly 50 percent incidence of exaggerated uterine activity with nipple stimulation although without any untoward event. A recent finding on this issue that nipple stimulation during pregnancy does not increase the plasma level "of oxytocin in the mother further confuses the position of the test (Kirschbaum, 1987).

In view of the above, most obstetricians now prefer to do the full six point non-stress assessment (as opposed to simple FM acceleration) supplemented by VAST instead of CST. Actually, logically, there is not much point in doing CST even for re-checking NST because both NST and CST have equal false positivity rate of 50 percent as mentioned above.

FETAL ACTOGRAM/ACTOCARDIOGRAM

The purpose of this equipment is to monitor full activity profile of the fetus (actography) including its limb movement, trunk movement and breathing movement during antepartum period along with continuous recording of its FHR pattern (actocardiography). Standard CTG machine, suitably modified, may be used for this purpose. No doubt this additional facility gives improved antenatal fetal monitoring.

Principle

The method uses the 'low frequency content' of the Doppler US signals of the FHR transducer to indicate fetal movement. In normal course of picking up heart beat by US these mild signals are discarded and all importance is given only to the strong signal coming from the fetal heart. But for the purpose of recording fetal activity, i.e. fetal movement monitoring, those mild signals, which represent the movement velocity below 4 cm/sec, are picked up and represented in the form of graph.

Mechanism

These modified and improved CTG machines give the activity profile of the fetus both in the form of graph and 'event mark'. It is so arranged in such machines that every time the graph amplitude goes above 40 percent of the full scale (a pre-set value), an 'Event mark' (a tiny black line) is printed along the top margin of toco channel (see Figs 13.49 and 13.50). Besides, these machines also give facility of choosing the 'frequency filter threshold' for printing the event marks of the range between zero to 99 percent. There is also arrangement for the events (movements) to make them audible.

Correlation

It has been found that with the event marker set at 40 percent filter threshold, in normal mature fetus, the sensitivity of actogram is 96 percent and its specificity is 68 percent when correlated with simultaneous real time US scan. Actogram, however, has not been found to be very useful during labor. (Sonicaid TEAM-User's Guide, 1996).

It is necessary to clarify here that, with the present technology, it is not yet possible to differentiate various types of movements (e.g. limb, trunk or breathing movement) from the actogram graph.

It should be noted that besides fetal movement—other types of movement such as maternal coughing, straining, even the transducer movement also do make peaks (humps and spikes) in the fetal movement graph.

Advantage

Actocardiograph can give a more precise biophysical profile of fetus than when it is done visually under US scanner and very much more easily. This investigation in conjunction with AFI (amniotic fluid index) gives a very reliable assessment of fetal health. To say the least, this automatic 'acto' facility gives the most reliable NST.

CTG ASSISTANCE IN DFMC BY MOTHER

CTG has an indispensable role to play for using the full predictive capability of daily fetal movement count by the mother. Here is to elaborate it further.

- As long as the movement is vigorous, count is high and mother is sure—one can do without CTG provided the clinical situation of the case does not demand it.
- But where the count is low or borderline or weak or faint and the mother is unsure about it—CTG assistance is a must. This is because of the large element of subjectivity involved in maternal count of FM—*a low count by the mother, on its own, cannot form an indication for interference* and hence each of such case must be evaluated by CTG.
- The other use of CTG lies in *training insensitive and unsure mothers* as to what is FM because it is well documented that mothers feel FM much better during a CTG monitoring session than otherwise.

Reasons for High Acceptance of Antenatal Fetal Monitoring by CTG

- It is objective
- It is non-invasive
- It is easy to perform—can be done by a nurse
- It involves far less handling of the patient in comparison to ultrasound scan. Once the two belts are fixed, no further handling is required.
- It is cheaper for the patient because –
    a. the machine is far less expensive than any other gadgetary monitoring device and
    b. because it can be used by junior level medical attendant—for making the tracing and also, with some training input, doing its preliminary reporting.
- It is easily repeated
- It is a bedside method
- Home monitoring is possible with great ease and advantage
- Easy telemetry facility through telephonic connection
- Reduces skilled manpower requirment leading to high productivity of the staff.

FURTHER READING

1. American College of Obst & Gyne (ACOG), Intrapartum Fetal Heart Monitoring, Practice Bulletin No. 70, December 2005.Quoted in William's Obstetrics, 23rd edition, 2010.
2. Arias F Practical Guide to High-risk Pregnancy and Delivery (2nd edn), St Louis: Mosby Year Book. 1993;3–20, 301–18, 413–29.
3. Arulkumaran S. In: Ratnam SS, Bhaskar Rao K, Arulkumaran S. Obstetrics and Gynaecology for Postgraduates, (1st edn). Chennai: Orient Longman. 1992;115–26.
4. Arulkumaran S, Montan S. Singapore Journal of Obstetrics and Gynaecology 1991;22(2):35–39.
5. Beard RW. Fetal heart rate patterns and their clinical interpretation. Bognor Regis, Sussex, UK: Sonicaid Ltd. 1974;l–56.
6. Cunningham FG, Mac Donald PC, Gant NF. William's Obstetrics, (19th edn). USA: Prentice Hall International Inc. 1993;1039.

7. Cunningham FG, Mac Donald PC, Gant NF, Leveno KJ, Gilstrap LC, Hankins GDV, Clark SL. Williams Obstetrics, (20th edn). USA: Prentice Hall International. 1997;364, 1009–22.

8. Cunningham FG, Leveno KJ, Bloom SL, et al, in William's Obstetrics, 23rd Edition, Intrapartum Assessment, Mc Graw Hill, New York, 2010;410–43.

9. Debdas AK, Kaur T. Abstract National Congress of Perinatology and Reproductive Biology. 6–10 February, Mumbai. 1986;5:23.

10. Debdas AK. Practical Cardiotocography. Published by Fetal Monitoring Research Centre, Jamshedpur, 1993;56–74.

11. Flynn AM, Kelly J. Recent Advances in Obst and Gynae. In: John Bonnar (Ed): Churchill Livingstone. 1982;14:25–45.

12. Freeman RK. Clinics in Perinatology 1982;9(2):265–70.

13. Fraser DM and Cooper MA in Myles Textbook for Midwives, 15th edition, Monitoring the Fetus, Churchill Livingstone, London, 2009;481–4

14. Hill WC, Moenning RK, Katz M, Kitzmiller JL. Obstet Gynecol 1984;64: 489–92.

15. Ingemarsson I, Ingemarsson E, Spencer JAD. Fetal Heart Rate Monitoring: A Practical Guide. Oxford: Oxford University Press. 1993;283–85.

16. Kirschbaum TH. In: Mishell DR, Kirschabaum TH, Morrow CP. Year Book of Obstetrics and Gynaecology. Chicago: Year Book Medical Publisher. 1987;143–78.

17. Magowan B, Owen P, Drife J: Clinical Obst Gynae, 2nd edition, Monitoring the Fetus in labor, Elsevier, Edinburg, 2009;331-43

18. Martin JH, Hamilton BE, Sutton PD, et al: in Births, Final data for 2002, National Vital Statistics Report, USA, Vol-52, No. 1, Haythsville MD, National Centre for Health Statistics, 2003

19. NICE (National Institute for Clinical Excellance) Guideline :The use of Electronic fetal monitoring: the use and interpretation of Cardiotocography in Intrapartum Fetal Surveillance, 2001, London

20. NICE (National Institute for Clinical Excellance) Guideline :The Clinical Guideline No. 70, Induction of labour, RCOG press, 2008, London

21. Read JA, Miller FC. Am J Obstet Gynecol 1977;129:512.

22. Sonicaid Team Fetal Monitor-User's guide: Publication No. 8909-8500, Issue-2,1, Kimber Road, Oxford, UK. 1996;70–73.

23. Steer PJ. Fetal heart rate patterns and their clinical interpretation. Sussex, UK: Oxford Sonicaid Ltd. 1986;1–44.

Uterine Activity— Normal and Abnormal

Techniques of doing tocography—both external and internal and the relative merits and demerits of each have already been described in detail earlier in Chapter-6 'Methods of Picking Up Uterine Activity: Tocography'. It is the actual clinical application of tocography and tocometry that is proposed to be discussed in this chapter.

However, it is recommended that the following clinically important headings should first be studied from Chapter-6 before starting this chapter:

1. Information that can be obtained from external tocography.
2. Drawbacks of external tocography.
3. Disadvantages of (fluid-filled) intrauterine catheter technique of internal tocometry.
4. Drawbacks of internal tocometry.
5. Place of internal tocometry.

CHARACTERISTICS OF UTERINE CONTRACTION

This will be discussed under the following headings:

- Frequency
- Duration
- Amplitude
- Basal tone
- Shape of the contraction curve.

Frequency of Contraction

Normal

- 1 in 10 mins at the beginning of labor.
- 2–3 in 10 mins—halfway through first stage.
- 5 in 10 mins towards the end of first stage and in second stage of labor.
  Frequency may reach 1 in 1 min towards the very end of second stage (Cunningham et al, 1989).

Abnormalities in Frequency

(in late first stage and second stage)
- Less than 5 in 10 mins—hypo/normal
- More than 5 in 10 mins—hyper.

Management of Abnormalities in Frequency

- Too frequent contraction
  - This almost invariably happens when contractions are stimulated artificially by Oxytocics to induce or augment. So, the Oxytocic should be reduced or stopped.
  - However, if in spite of frequent contractions labor is not progressing satisfactorily and there is no fetal or maternal distress—oxytocin drip has to be given under CTG control after exclusion of obstruction to the passage of delivery.
    Since frequent contraction can cause fetal hypoxia—these cases need electronic fetal monitoring.
- Infrequent contraction
  These cases need oxytocin infusion under CTG control.
  Doses – To be determined by titration and should be sufficient to augment uterine activity to—maximum 5 in 10 mins and upto maximum 8 μ/min dose.

Note

If the labor is progressing satisfactorily, i.e. there is progressive dilatation and descent—infrequent contraction need not be treated.

Duration of Contraction

Normal—30 to 60 sec. in first stage, can go upto 90 sec. in second stage (Cunningham et al, 1989).

Abnormality

Prolonged contraction—It, usually, is the result of hyperstimulation with oxytocic and hence, its management will be to switch off or reduce oxytocin.

Short lived contraction—

- Here one has to ascertain whether the patient is really in labor or not.
- Such patients need oxytocin drip or Prostaglandin tablet/ Misoprostol vaginally or sublingually, provided there is no contraindication and the dose of oxytocin has to be titrated with the help of CTG-on the frequency of contraction and the state of FHR.

  If the membranes are intact it may have to be ruptured.

Amplitude

This is determined by measuring intrauterine pressure.

Normal

First stage

- Range—20 to 60 mm of Hg, may go upto 75 mm
- Dilatation pressure—starts at 20 mm
- Pain pressure—starts at 25 mm (Dewhurst, 1981)

Second stage

With combined force of uterine contraction and maternal bearing down effort the pressure may rise upto 150 mm or more (Ingemarsson et al, 1993).

Abnormality

- Hypotonic—Peak pressure less than 30 mm

- Hypertonic—Peak pressure more than 70 mm.
- The amplitude of uterine activity is also expressed in KPas. The normal levels of uterine activity as expressed in this unit are—from 700 KPas/15 mins to 1500 KPas/15 mins (Steer, 1986).

Management of Abnormality of Amplitude of Contraction

- Hypotonic cases—Oxytocic in titrated dosage.
- Hypertonic cases—Needs close observation of fetal and maternal condition, to be acted upon depending on the condition found of these.

  In both the instances any obstruction must be excluded.

  In hypertonic cases abruption of placenta must be kept in mind. If the patient is on Oxytocic—it must be stopped.

  In some cases instant tocolysis may have to be done by giving Terbutalin 0.25 mg subcuteneously.

Note

Recently, fetal cerebral blood flow study on real time with the help of near infra-red spectroscopy (NIRS) done in second stage during Valsalva (i.e. on the face of additive effect of uterine power and maternal bearing down effort) has shown occurrence of reduction of -

a. oxyhemoglobin level,
b. oxygen index and
c. oxygen saturation in fetal brain even in normal second stage of labor (Aldrich et al, 1995).

Basal Uterine Tone

This means the intrauterine pressure in between contractions, i.e. during uterine quiescence.

- Normal—In normal labor it varies between 8 and 12 mm of Hg.
- Abnormal—Basal tone higher than 20 mm is considered as definitely pathological because it can lead to fetal distress by constricting the arterioles at the placental bed. If the patient is on oxytocic it should be reduced or stopped.

Shape of the Contraction Curve

Though two shapes of the curve have been described called type A and type B, these are of no clinical importance. The only abnormality of shape that should cause concern is—double peaked or triple peaked contraction because this, in effect, is equivalent to a prolonged contraction which means prolonged constriction of retroplacental vessels and consequent fetal hypoxia (See **Fig. 13.35**—'Uterine polysystole').

Units of Measurement of Uterine Power

Montevideo Unit

This is calculated as—Amplitude × Frequency over 10 min. period.

Alexandria Unit

This is calculated as—Mean amplitude × Frequency × Mean duration of contraction over 10 min. period.

The difference between the above two units:

- While Montavideo unit does not take into account the 'duration' of contraction Alexandria unit does. So, it is an improvement but is more complicated to calculate.
- Some new terms used to express uterine activity e.g. Uterine Activity Integral (UAI).
- Even the area of contraction can be calculated electronically. These are of theoretical interest.

Clinical Correlation of Uterine Contraction with Intrauterine Pressure

- Uterine contractions become clinically palpable – only when it raises the intrauterine pressure above 10 mm of Hg.
- Mother feels pain – only when the contraction raises the intrauterine pressure to above 15 mm of Hg. So, it may be called – the pain pressure.

    Since a minimum of this amount of pressure is required to attempt distending of lower uterine segment and cervix – it may be called the *dilatation pressure*.

No attempt should be made to try and depress the uterine wall with fingers during a contraction to assess the intensity of contraction. It is useless and also unkind.

The 'Reality' of Uterine Contraction Monitoring

Only two parameters of uterine contraction need monitoring to be of benefit – the
- Frequency and
- Duration of contraction.

This gives idea not only about the prospect of progress but also whether placental perfusion is getting affected or not—by too frequent and too prolonged contractions and through that the possibility of occurrence of fetal distress.

These can be easily done by patient's attendant or even by the mother herself.

Relation of Uterine Contraction with the Position of the Patient

Supine position

Contractions in this position comes more frequently but they are of lower amplitude and hence are less effective and more disturbing to the mother. Apart from causing supine hypotension, this is another reason for advicing patient to avoid supine position during labor.

Lateral Position

Contraction in this position come at greater interval but are more strong and hence more effective.

Erect Position

Characters of contraction in this position are same as that of lateral position.

Difference in Character of Contraction between Spontaneous and Induced or Augmented Labor

The main difference is (as has been found out by intrauterine pressure measurement and also taking into account the frequency and duration of contraction) there occurs '*generation of greater pressure*' in induced labor in comparison to spontaneous labor (Ingemarsson et al, 1993). There occurs much higher rate of polysystoles, i.e.

>5 contractions in 10 minutes (Nama and Arulkumaran, 2009).

Obesity and Uterine Contractility

Obese women, i.e. those with high BMI show poor uterine contractillity. In vitro experiment suggest that elevated cholesterol may cause disruption of signalling mechanism (Zhang et al, 2007)

PRACTICAL APPROACH TO TOCOMETRY IN LABOR

1. The best method of assessing uterine power is to *assess its effects* namely:

    a. *The cervimetric progress of labor*

    b. *The absence of fetal distress*

    If the cervix is dilating satisfactorily, presenting part is descending steadily and FHR is remaining normal—contraction, whatever may be its character, can be regarded as normal.

    On the other hand, if dilatation is slow (on an average less than 1 cm /hour) or is arrested and/or FHR is showing signs of distress—the contraction should be regarded as abnormal—(for that particular case) whatever palpatory or tocographic evaluation may show.

2. As a corollary to above, it may be concluded that monitoring of the different features of uterine contraction, like its frequency, duration, amplitude, shape of the trace, basal tone, etc. is not really the best method of assessing uterine power because

    i. These vary even normally from patient to patient and

    ii. Abnormalities of these may not necessarily hinder dilatation of cervix or cause fetal distress.

3. None of those peculiar types of abnormal uterine action like— colicky uterus, asymmetrical uterine contraction, reversed polarity, etc. described in some text books can be diagnosed *even by standard internal tocometry* procedure using 'one' intrauterine catheter. So, they are really simply research findings. In any case, treatment of all these abnormality of uterine action is oxytocin infusion unless it is contraindicated or unless these have been caused by oxytocin itself.

Note

If the cervix has dilated satisfactorily but the presenting part has not descended one should look for cause either in the passenger (e.g. occipito-posterior position, big baby, etc.) or in the passage (pelvic capacity) or both and should not try to augment uterine contraction by oxytocin infusion

Total Uterine Activity – A Simple Phenomenon and Logic

It is a reflection *of the resistance* that cervical and pelvic tissues put up against fetal descent. This explains why primis require much more number of contractions and takes much longer to deliver in comparison to multi.

TOCOLYSIS

This means lysing uterine contraction for therapeutic reasons.

Scope of Use of CTG for Tocolysis

CTG is definitely required for doing scientific and objective tocolysis for the following vital purpose -

- In order to objectively establish that the case needs tocolysis, i.e. to establish that the pain of the patient is actually due to uterine contractions, i.e. she is truly in premature labor

- For titrating the dose of the tocolytic drug
- For terminating the tocolytic therapy.

Indication of Tocolysis

- To stop premature onset of labor
  (**To label a case as one of premature labor there has to be 'documented' contraction of at least 4 in 20 min or 8 in 60 min frequency, i.e. one contraction in every 5 to 7.5 mins).**
- Exaggerated uterine contraction producing signs of fetal distress
- Cord prolapse to alley cord compression—while arranging cesarean section.
- For doing external cephalic version (Cunningham et al, 2010) [Non-CTG use—to facilitate reposition of uterus in cases of postpartum inversion of uterus].

Contraindications of Tocolysis

Cardiac disease, eclampsia and severe pre-eclampsia, intrauterine infection, intrauterine fetal death, placenta praevia and abruption of placenta.

FURTHER READING

1. Aldrich CJ, D'Antona D, Spencer JAD, Wyatt JS, Peebles DM, Delpy DT, et al. Brit J Obstet Gynaecol 1995;102:448–53.
2. American College of Obst & Gyne (ACOG), Intrapartum Fetal Heart Monitoring, Practice Bulletin No. 70, December 2005. Quoted in William's Obstetrics, 23rd edition, 2010.
3. Cunningham FG, Mac Donald PC, Gant NF. William's Obstetrics, (18th edn), USA: Prentice-Hall International Inc. 1989;213–6, 290–305.
4. Cunningham FG, Gant NF, Leveno KJ, et al. William's Obstetrics, (21st edn), New York: McGraw Hill. 2001;530,643,716–7,796.
5. Dewhurst J. Integrated Obstetrics and Gynaecology for Post Graduates, (3rd edn). Blackwell Scientific Publications. 1981;108–10,180–1.
6. Ingemarsson I, Ingemarsson E, Spencer JAD. Fetal heart rate monitoring: A practical guide. Oxford: Oxford University Press. 1993;34–49.

7. Magowan B, Owen P, Drife J: Clinical Obst Gynae, 2nd edition, Monitoring the Fetus in labor, Elsevier, Edinburg, 2009;349–54

8. Morrison JJ. Progress in Obstetrics and Gynaecology: In: John Studd (Ed): London: Churchill Livingstone. 1996;12:67–86.

9. Myles Textbook for Midwives:Edited by Fraser DM and Cooper MA, Monitoring the Fetus, Church Livingstone, London, 15th edition, 2009;461–463, 481–4

10. Nama V and Arulkumaran S: 'Uterine Contractions' in the book Best Practice in Labor and Delivery, Edited by Warren R and Arulkumaran S, 2009;54–65

11. Sonicaid TEAM Fetal monitor—User's guide: Publication No. 8909-8500, Issue-2, 1, Kimber Road, Oxford, UK. 1996;54,63–69.

12. Steer PJ. Fetal heart rate patterns and their clinical interpretation. Sussex, UK: Oxford Sonicaid Ltd. 1986;1–44.

13. William's Obstetrics: 23rd edition, Edited by Cunningham FG, Leveno KJ, Bloom SL, Hauth JC, Rouse DJ and Spong CY, Intrapartum Assessment, Mc Graw Hill, New York, 2010;410–43.

14. Zhang J, Bricker Lwray Squenby S : Poor uterine contractility in obese women, Br J Obstet Gynecol, 2007;114:343–8.

Applied Cardiotocography— Intranatal

The Pressing Need for Fetal Monitoring in Labor

The three unique stress factors for fetus during labor are:

- Factor of uterine contraction
- Factor of head compression
- Factor of possible cord stress.

Factor of Uterine Contraction

Physiologically, labor is recognized as the most stressful period for the fetus out of its nine months of intrauterine life. This is because during this period its blood supply gets cut off temporarily and fractionally with every contraction of the uterus because this happens to partially obstruct the blood vessels going to the placenta through the criss-cross muscle fibres of myometrium. It has been shown by internal cardiotocography and tocometry that inter-villous blood supply does not get affected until the amplitude of contraction exceeds 30 mm Hg (Steer, 1986). Doppler studies provide even more objective evidences.

So much about the placental blood flow, let us now see what happens to the *oxygenation and blood supply of the fetal brain* during an uterine contraction. This is what has been found about these most vital parameters (since it is related to the question of brain damage) by Near Infrared Spectroscopy (NIRS) done during pushing in second stage of labor (Aldrich et al, 1995).

De-oxy Hb	-	↑ by 0.79 micromol/100 gm of brain
Oxy Hb	-	↓ by 0.19 micromol/100 gm of brain
Cerebral O_2 index	-	↓ by 1.00 micromol/100 gm of brain
Cerebral O_2 saturation	-	↓ by 9 percent
Cerebral blood vol	-	↑ by 0.33 ml/100 gm of brain

However, in spite of the above slightly worrying picture nothing untoward happens to the fetus if it is healthy, if the labor contractions are normal and if the placenta has adequate reserve.

Fetal distress, birth asphyxia, brain damage, intrauterine fetal death, hypoxic neonatal death, etc. are likely to occur only -

a. If the fetus is already compromised antenatally—when, even the normal uterine contractions can precipitate distress, or

b. If the uterine contractions are exaggerated—when, even a perfectly healthy fetus having an efficient placenta may be affected. This is purely contraction related problem, which is peculiar to labor, can occur:

- As a result of undetected Oxytocin or Prostaglandin over-stimulation, e.g. as in the course of induction or acceleration of labor, or

- As a consequence of some abnormalities in the mechanical component of labor like some sort of obstruction to the passage of delivery.

Factor of Head Compression

Some degree of head compression is inevitable and is normal during normal labor. However, excessive compression specially over a long period causing supermoulding as can happen in presence of obstruction constitutes neurological stress for the fetus and demands close FH monitoring.

Factor of Possible Cord Stress

It is well known that most cord associated problems like cord stretching, cord entrapment between the own body parts of the fetus, cord prolapse, cord presentation and cord entanglements—whether occult or overt—become apparent and exert their deleteries effect on fetus only during labor—a secondary effect of uterine contractions.

PROBLEM OF CLINICAL METHODS OF FETAL MONITORING IN LABOR

1. Fetal hypoxia is 'silent' in its appearance and infliction. So, its detection calls for recurrent auscultation of FH at short intervals over long period (10–18 hours) which is tedious and physically laborious.

2. It demands *'one-to-one'* *'skilled'* manning which is very difficult to accomplish and also expensive (perpetual expense towards the salary and perks of the staff).

3. For early detection of fetal distress—the auscultation must necessarily be done "during" (right through) contraction which is impossible both by a stethoscope and even by Doptone because during contraction FH tends to go out of focus from US beam. FHR counting soon after a contraction is also quite difficult and need very high skill and commitment.

4. There is no means of assessing 'amplitude' of uterine contraction and also hypertonic and hypotonic state by clinical examination (possible only by internal tocometry).

5. By simple auscultation fetal distress is diagnosed either too promptly and loosely or too late because of lack of objectivity and precision.

6. Since it is not objective—the findings always remain questionable. One has to believe somebody's findings.

7. Clinical monitoring also lacks the strength of uniformity and hard scientific proof.

8. It is heavily-dependent on human factors like human lapses, error, sincerity, honesty—even the physical and mental state

(fatigue, overwork, etc.) of the observer.
(Also see Chapter 32—"Place of CTG Today").

How CTG can Help to Overcome the Above Problem?

CTG, in fact, can remove all the above problems of clinical monitoring. However, the main contribution of CTG lies in the following areas:

- Its ability to precisely record the main stresser, i.e. the uterine contraction
- Its ability to record FHR right through contraction
- Its ability to detect two very important and reliable signs of fetal distress—the late deceleration and poor baseline variability which are not possible to spot clinically
- Its ability to provide hard evidence (the paper-tracing) of the events which can be very useful for medicolegal purpose in case of claim-suit
- Its capacity to exclude the problems related to human factor as mentioned
- Its ability to reduce manpower (one-to-one skilled manning) while improving the quality and precision of monitoring
- Its ability to allow distant monitoring and ambulatory monitoring.

Changing Trend in the Use of CTG for Intrapartum Fetal Monitoring

Trends of Seventies

"Monitor all—and all through labor": In seventies, charged by enthusiasm for the new and also by the urge for hard objectivity the trend had been to monitor and manage 'all' labors by cardiotocography irrespective of whether the fetus was of high-risk or low-risk category. Probably the philosophy behind such action was—every fetus is precious and hence should be monitored in most precise manner.

Trends of Eighties

"Don't monitor all – monitor only the high-risk cases": In eighties, as more and more results of large scale studies of the use of intrapartum CTG were available and as more and more experiences were gained about the limitations of the method, conclusions like this started emerging:

a. It is much too expensive to monitor all labors,

b. It is unnecessary to monitor all labors electronically because it entails too much work for too little real benefit since only a very small proportion is found to show abnormality,

c. CTG monitoring of low-risk or normal cases often increases the cesarean section rate without any corresponding reduction in perinatal mortality.

So, on the basis of above disquieting findings the new consensus that emerged in eighties was—CTG should be used only for the management of labor of high-risk cases and not all cases, the risks, for the above purpose, were broadly defined as follows:

The risk classification

1. All cases of 'Bad obstetric history' (BOH) where the mishap can be linked to fetal hypoxia, e.g. cases with history of stillbirth, low Apgar baby, respiratory distress syndrome, neonatal death and spastic child in previous pregnancy.

2. All high premium babies as in:
   • Elderly mothers
   • Diabetic mothers
   • Cases with history of long infertility and, of course, IVF fetuses,
   • Cases with history of recurrent abortion

3. All cases where fetus is likely to be potentially hypoxic like:
   • All IUGR cases
   • All post-dated pregnancy cases
   • All cases of hypertensive disorder

- All induced labor cases (they are high risk in any case)
- All meconium stained liquor cases
- All cases of prolonged or static labor

4. All cases on continuous epidural analgesia (see Chapter 24) because of its potential of causing maternal hypotension which has known deleterious effect on fetus and also because these blocking drugs have direct depressant effect on fetal myocardium. Besides here, labor being totally painless—uterine contraction are a bit difficult to assess clinically and are best monitored by a machine.

5. Non-obstetric indication—VIP patients.

Problems with the 'Risk Approach'

- A high percentage of perinatal problems occur in the so-called 'no risk' or ' low-risk' cases (see below).
- How can one withhold an improved facility when it is readily available right in the labor room.
- How to face a couple and their lawyer if something happens to an unmonitored (by CTG) 'low-risk' case.

Trends of Nineties

"Monitor all – but only on admission in labor and just for 20 minutes":
In nineties, the trend seem to have reversed again in favor of the old, i.e. in favor of CTG covering of all labors but this time not wishfully but on very sound and logical ground with both science and economics in view as detailed below:

Screen and assess each and every fetus cardiotocographically 'for a short period' of about 20 mins right on admission in labor to determine, from the nature of the tracing, the specific monitoring requirement of that particular fetus both in terms of:

- Intensity of monitoring, i.e. whether the case should be further monitored
  - clinically or
  - cardiotocographically and also
- Duration and Frequency of monitoring, i.e. whether the case should be covered by CTG

— continuously or

— intermittently

and this is what is called Admission test (Arulkumaran, 1992) (See later in this chapter for details about this test).

This ingeneous approach would appear to ensure maximum utilization of CTG machine for the most deserving cases and thereby offer maximum fetal safety to them. Not only this – this regime would also effectively screen all the low risk cases as well,

So, in effect, this system would cover *all* cases and with not a great deal of extra investment.

The logistics for (also) screening the no risk (actually there is no such entity as no risk) or low-risk cases are:

• Even after rigorous selection based on known antenatal risk classification (as mentioned above)—fetal morbidity and mortality do occur in the so-called low-risk group as well as evidenced in the following reports.

• Incidence of acidosis at birth has not been found to be *very* different between low-risk and high-risk population (Arulkumaran, 1992).

• Fifty percent of neonatal abnormalities has been found to occur in low risk pregnancies. (Stone and Murray, 1995).

Trends of CTG Monitoring of this Millennium

"Double check all pathological trace by a second more objective method": The logic for introduction of double checking is – as high as 50 percent cases of pathological trace do not show fetal acidosis and also these babies are born with good Apgar score. Methods of double-checking an abnormal or non-reassuring CTG trace that are currently available are:

• VAST(see Chapter No. 19)

• F-ECG (see Chapter No. 21)

• Scalp Stimulation Test (see later in this chapter)

• Fetal Pulse Oxymetry (see Chapter No. 23)

• Micro FBS and instant Lactate assay (see Chapter No. 23).

ADMISSION TEST (ADMISSION CTG TEST)

As described above—it is a dynamic screening test for the state of oxygenation of fetus right on admission of the mother into labor room, i.e. more or less at the beginning of labor. This test proposes to assess the placental reserve by checking the hypoxic (or otherwise) response of fetal heart during the phase of temporary occlusion of the retroplacental blood vessels brought about by the physiological stress of repeated uterine contraction. The test this way assesses the ability of the fetus to withstand the hypoxic stress of the process of labor.

Procedure

After full history taking and examination CTG leads are put on the patient and the machine is run on for 15–20 minutes just as in NST. The duration of monitoring may be reduced to 10 minutes if, even within that very short period the tracing shows normal baseline FHR, normal baseline variability, 2 accelerations of 15 BPM lasting for 15 seconds and 2 contractions without any deceleration (see later 'Admission test with fetal acoustic stimulation').

Observation and Plan of Management on the Admission Tracing

Broadly in practical terms, depending upon its particular feature, any tracing can be allocated into one of these three categories:
- Absolutely normal trace
- Grossly abnormal trace
- Suspicious or equivocal trace

The recommended plan of management of each of these category is described below.

Absolutely Normal Trace

If the admission tracing is normal in every way—it can be predicted that the chance of this fetus developing hypoxia in next 5 hours or so is unlikely apart from that due to unpredictable acute events (Ingemarsson et al, 1986). Hence, these cases can be monitored clinically with intermittent (every 30 min.) FH auscultation (preferably soon after a contraction) by fetoscope or better still by doptone for next 4 hours when another short strip of CTG (of 10 to 15 mins duration) may be taken. According to Arulkumaran 1992, if 'Admission test' was normal, a gradually developing hypoxia would be reflected by a gradually rising baseline FHR which should be detectable by ordinary auscultation. So, in the event of such a case developing tachycardia the case should be checked by CTG forthwith.

However, presence of meconium even in these cases with absolutely normal trace makes the patient a candidate for continuous CTG monitoring.

Grossly Abnormal Trace

If the tracing shows more than two elements of CTG abnormality, e.g. poor baseline variability, baseline tachycardia plus late deceleration—arrangement should be made for immediate delivery of the fetus. However, if facilities are available *in the same CTG machine*, F-ECG with STAN software, it should be switched on to see whether the fetal myocardium is also showing signs of hypoxia or not. Doing a prompt fetal blood sampling (FBS) to check whether the fetus is acidotic or not is a good proposition but is too complex. It is noteworthy that Beard (1974) found only around 50 percent incidence of acidosis in fetal blood sample even with severe CTG abnormality.

In author's view fetuses with such severe abnormality is better delivered straightaway—may be before acidosis develops.

Suspicious Trace/Equivocal Trace

If the tracing shows just one or two abnormal CTG parameters—the case should be monitored continuously for further development towards better or worse while instituting the usual corrective measures like—turning the patient on her side, stopping oxytocic, giving oxygen inhalation etc. But, ideally, in these cases the condition of the fetus should be checked by another method like—FBS, FAST or possibly by scalp stimulation test. In author's unit, FAST is used for this purpose. Arulkumaran (1992) found only 10 percent of fetuses of this category to develop 'fetal distress' as defined by the necessity to institute operative delivery for fetal distress and by the birth of the baby with Apgar's 5 at 1 min (see also Chapter No. 22 "Non-re-assuring CTG trace").

However, if the liquor is meconium stained with such a tracing, the baby should be delivered immediately.

It is necessary to emphasize that the result of all admission tests must be interpreted with full clinical picture of the patient and then acted upon.

Recent Report on the Value of Admission Test

Metaanalysis of available trials suggest that mothers with Admission CTG were more likely to have epidural analgesia, continuous electronic fetal monitoring and fetal blood sampling and instrumental birth (Bix, Reiner, Klovning et al, 2005).

Antenatal care in developed countries, the fetuses at risk of developing hypoxia on the face of stress of labor contractions are generally get picked up antenatally by serial ultrasound scan, Doppler, etc. precluding the need for Admission test.

However, it may have role in busy obstetric units like those with >10,000 deliveries/year and has limited resources (Edwin and Arulkumaran, 2008)

PLACE OF 'VAST' IN LABOR

Vibroacoustic stimulation test (VAST) can be used in labor for the following two purposes:
• As an 'Admission test'
• As an alternative to FBS
  (see the exclusive chapter on the subject: Chapter No. 19)

SCALP STIMULATION TEST

This simple instant test is under investigation with encouraging results.

Methods of Scalp Stimulation

- *By applying a gentle pinch* by a traumatic Allis tissue forceps on the fetus's scalp: In author's view pinching scalp with Allis tissue forceps to stimulate the fetus is a bit too drastic and unkind because this causes severe pain to the fetus as can be easily demonstrated by applying the same forceps-pinch on baby's scalp soon after its birth. The act makes the baby scream incessantly and to pitiably throw its limbs in the air. Presumably same thing happens when it is done when the baby is still in utero and this may severely stress the baby and may make it to inhale liquor which may even be meconium stained. It should never be done.

- *By applying firm digital pressure on fetus scalp:* In fact, this *Digital pressure method* is sometimes automatically gets done during vaginal examination in labor while exploring the surface of the head to locate the various sutures and fontanelles in order to find the correct position of the head in relation to various quadrants of pelvis.

  It should also be remembered that too firm pressure on fetal head may cause fetal bradycardia rather than acceleration (see **Fig. 17.1**).

Experimental Evidence about the Validity of Scalp Stimulation Test

Clark et al (1984) subjected each of their 100 patients showing heart tracings suggestive of fetal hypoxia to both the above form of stimulation—'pressure' followed by 'pinch' just prior to scalp blood sampling for pH. They found that those fetuses which responded to the above stimulation by acceleration of their FHR by 15 BPM lasting for at least 15 seconds had pH—equal to or more than 7.19 which constituted 50 percent of their patients. Significance of lack of acceleration i.e. negative test was however inconclusive.

From the above study the authors concluded that such stimulation test with positive response can reduce the necessity for scalp blood sampling by approximately 50 percent in the presence of abnormal FH tracing on standard CTG.

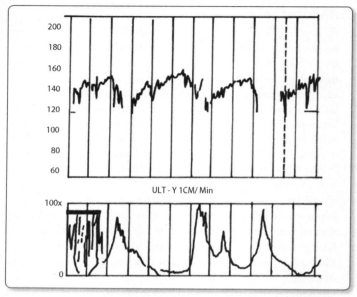

Fig. 17.1 This is a tracing of typical type I dip or early deceleration. Notice that the deceleration has 'started early' in contraction and recovered before the contraction is over. Also notice that the lowest point of deceleration has exactly coincided with the peak of uterine contraction. The important thing here is—the baseline FHR and baseline variability of FHR is preserved. This patient was fully dilated with head deep in the pelvis. Notice that the third dip was of greater magnitude than the first two dips. This was produced by finger pressure on head during PV during that particular contraction exaggerating the head compression and thereby aggravating the deceleration

Indication of Use of Scalp Stimulation Test

- *As a routine* during normal vaginal examination in labor as an additional evidence of fetal 'Wellness'.
- As a *double-check procedure* in the case already showing some CTG signs of fetal compromise (see **Figs 13.37** to **13.39**).
- As an *alternative to fetal blood sampling* in the second group of cases in the units where such facilities are available.

Drawback

Repeated vaginal examination to perform scalp stimulation test may introduce infection.

SPECIAL FEATURES OF CTG MONITORING IN SECOND STAGE

Please see the exclusive chapter on this – 'Special Features of CTG of Second Stage of Labor', Chapter 33.

SOME UNUSUAL CAUSES OF DECELERATION DURING LABOR

In labor, episodes of deceleration have been reported under the following unexpected situations:

* During micturition while sitting on a bed pan
* During maternal vomiting (Beard, 1971; Ingemarsson et al, 1993).

Two possible reasons have been suggested as the cause of this unusual phenomenon:

a. Marked rise in intrauterine pressure that occurs during these activities perhaps causes temporary reduction in uteroplacental perfusion.

b. Transient marked compression of fetal head stimulating fetal vagal centre.

The other unusual situations where deceleration may be seen in CTG tracing are:

* Application of digital pressure on fetal head during examination
* During application of scalp electrode
* During insertion of intrauterine catheter.

In all these instances, it is the vagal reflex which is responsible for such occurrence and not hypoxia.

FURTHER READING

1. Aldrich CJ, D'Antona D, Spencer J AD, Wyatt JS, Peebles DM, Delpy DT, Reynolds EOR. Br J Obstet Gynaecol 1995;102:448–53.
2. Arias F. Practical Guide to High Risk Pregnancy and Delivery, (2nd edn), St Louis: Mosby Year Book, 1993;413–29.
3. Arulkumaran S. Ratnam SS, Bhaskar Rao K, Arulkumaran S (Eds). Obstetrics and Gynaecology for Postgraduates, (1st edn). Madras, India: Orient Longman Ltd, 1992;115–26.
4. Bix E, Reiner LM, Klovning A et al: Prognostic value of labor Admission Test and its effectiveness compared with auscultation only: a systematic review, BJOG, 2005;112:1595–604.
5. Beard RW, Fillshie GM, Knight CA, Roberts GM. J Obstet Gynaecol Br Cwlth; 1971;78:865–81.
6. Beard RW F, et al. Heart rate patterns and their clinical interpretation, Bognor Regis, Sussex, UK: Sonicaid Ltd., 1974;1–56.
7. Clerk SL, Gimovsky ML, Miller FC. Am J Obstet Gynecol 1984;148:274.
8. Edwin C and Arulkumaran S: Electronic Fetal Heart Monitoring in current & future practice, The Journal of O & G of India, 2008;58:121–30.
9. Ingemarsson I, Arulkumaran S, Ingemarsson E, Tambyraja RI, Ratnam SS. Obstet Gynecol 1986;68:800–06.
10. Ingemarsson I, Ingemarsson E and Spencer JAD. Fetal Heart Rate Monitoring—A Practical Guide. Oxford: Oxford University Press, 1993;41.
11. Spencer JAD. Brit J Obstet Gynaecol 100: Supplement 1993;9:4–7.
12. Steer PJ. Fetal heart rate patterns and their clinical interpretation, Sussex, UK: Oxford Sonicaid Ltd., 1986;1–44.
13. Stone PR, Murray HG. John Bonnar (Ed). Recent Advances in Obst and Gynae, Vol-19, London: Churchill Livingstone, 1995;45–62.
14. William's Obstetrics: 23rd edition, Edited by Cunningham FG, Leveno KJ, Bloom SL, Hauth JC, Rouse DJ and Spong CY, Intrapartum Assessment, Mc Graw Hill, New York, 2010;410-43.

Fetal Sleep, Rest, Activity and CTG

A clear understanding of these is required in order to be able to interpret CTG tracings correctly. This has been discussed below under two broad headings—antenatal and intranatal.

I – DURING THE ANTENATAL PERIOD

Some mothers complain that sometime the baby does not move at all for hours. We don't know how to explain that, but what we know through studies by CTG that, like neonates and adults, fetuses also do rest and sleep and certainly during the antenatal period.

Four Levels of Fetal Activity and Sleep

Existence of these have been fairly clearly recognised in third trimester specially in last four intrauterine weeks (Ingemarsson et al, 1993) comprising of two-sleep-like levels (Steer, 1986) and two levels of wakefulness. These are as follows:

Deep Sleep-like State

This is like the sleep 'without rapid eye movement (REM)' as can be observed in a neonate. In this fetal state mother does not feel any fetal movement. CTG done during this period shows very low baseline variability (around 5-bpm—even less) and no FH acceleration and hence may worry obstetrician. This is also an eminent cause of false positive non-stress test (NST).

Hence, if one happens to catch this fetal state—one should continue CTG monitoring for 40 or 50 minutes by which time in a healthy fetus this sleep cycle should be, almost invariably, over and the fetus will show normal FH variation, normal movement (may be little excessive movement) and good FM acceleration. It is noteworthy that sometimes this deep sleep-like state may last for, as long as, 90 minutes during labour. However, it is best to be cautious if variability does not return by 40 minutes.

To save time, money and immobilisation of patient and also to allay anxiety, one can do a VAST, i.e. give a vibroacoustic stimulation to the fetus (see the exclusive chapter on this—the Chapter 19) to break the sleep cycle and observe the instant FH and FM response. A fetus not responding to VAST should be considered compromised.

Light Sleep-like State

This sleep is comparable to neonatal REM sleep. In this sleep-state mother may feel only rare occasional FM. CTG done in this phase show normal baseline variability but rare (FM) acceleration.

Quiet Awake State

As the term implies, this state is comparable with neonatal quiet awake state. In this, CTG trace would show normal baseline variability and at least two FM acceleration in twenty minutes.

Active Awake State

This is usually seen at the end of deep sleep or after stimulation. CTG done at this state shows lot of movements, which mother also confirms, and there is good acceleration with each movement. Sometimes, there occurs such a lot of movement with FH acceleration that one acceleration merges into another producing a short episode of baseline tachycardia which soon settles.

This cycle of sleep and wakefulness continues even during labor.

CTG Cycling

The presence of the above oscillation in CTG trace of 'Active' and 'quiet' epochs constitutes the basis of introduction of the term *'CTG cycling'* and is considered as a sign of **healthy** fetal state. "Cycling should be present to declare neurologically normal behavioral state (Arulkumaran, 2012)".

II - DURING LABOR

Does the fetus sleep during the process of labor?
Can the fetus sleep during the process of labor?

Intrauterine Fetal Environment during Labor

Un-nerving Natural Disturbances

- Recurrent turmoil in the liquor pool
- Recurrent squeeze and squash on its body
- Constant and increasing compression on its head
- Occasional stretch and pull on its life-cord

All these are occasioned by inevitable incessant uterine contractions.

Disturbance Created by Man Initiated Caring Endeavor

- Repeated abdominal manipulation / palpation specially that of its head – causing sore head
- Repeated prodding on its spine by the fetoscope.
- Repeated stimulation of its scalp if not its skull by repeated vaginal examination.
- Repeated hitting of its heart by ultrasonic beam in case it is being monitored by Doptone, more so by the US FH transducer of CTG machine
- Prolonged sting by two needles (the scalp electrodes) stuck on its head—in case it is being monitored by internal method of CTG
- Intermittent tickle here and there on its body by the intrauterine catheter if that has been used

• Constant irritation by the oxymetry probe – if that has been used However, surprisingly, studies have shown that it probably can and does sleep (due to biologically programmed Endorphin secretion). The cycle of sleep and wakefulness do continue during labor.

HOW TO EXCLUDE FETAL SLEEP BY CTG

Necessity for Embarking into such an Action

In a case having antenatal CTG—if the baseline variability is found to be very low, i.e. 'less than 5-bpm' (i e if CTG is found to be flat) and there is also total absence of FM and FM acceleration – the state lasting for more than 40 minutes – it is possible that the fetus is in 'deep sleep-like state' provided other pathological causes for it can be excluded.

Management of Such a Trace

a. Firstly, the clinical situation of the case should be critically reviewed to exclude or establish the following conditions which can also produce such a trace:
   • Any factor which could cause fetal hypoxia, e.g. IUGR, oligo-hydramnios, etc.
   • Any possibility of fetal CNS malformation
   • Any sedation given to mother and, for a case in labor
   • Whether the liquor is meconium stained or not.

b. If these are not present then the patient may be given a vibro-acoustic stimulation and FH and FM response observed (see Chapter 19—Vibroacoustic Stimulation Test-VAST) or

c. Alternatively the monitoring session may be extended upto 50–90 minutes to see whether the activity cycle returns or not.

FURTHE READING

1. Arulkumaran S : Obstetrician at fault with CTG Interpretation, Proceedings of AICOG 1012, Varanasi, January 27–30, 2012, Federation of Obstetrics & Gynaecology Societies of India, p 11.

2. Debdas AK. Practical Cardiotocography (1st edn). New Delhi: Jaypee Brothers Medical Publishers. 1998;82–83.

3. D'Souza R and Arulkumaran S. 'Intrapartum Fetal Surveillance' in the book Best Practice in Labor and Delivery, Edited by Warren R and Arulkumaran S, 2009;38–53.

4. Ingemarsson I, Ingemarsson E, Spencer JADF, et al. Heart Rate Monitoring—A special guide. Oxford: Oxford University Press. 1993;283–85.

5. Steer PJ. Fetal heart rate patterns and their clinical interpretations. Sussex, UK:Oxford Sonicaid Ltd. 1986;1–44.

6. Strachan B. 'The Management of intrapartum Fetal Distress' in the book Best Practice in Labor and Delivery, Edited by Warren R and Arulkumaran S, 2009;66–75

Fetal Vibroacoustic Stimulation Test (VAST) by CTG

This fetal surveillance test aims to assess the functional state of fetal CNS and its reflex cardiovascular response and through these its blood oxygen status. It is a test for relatively acute fetal distress and, may also help the obstetrician to discover unsuspected cases of chronic fetal distress. This test has been quoted as the most commonly used antepartum fetal surveillance test (Arias, 1993).

BASIS OF VAST

The test is based on the following observations:

The finding that fetal cochlear apparatus gets mature enough to appreciate acoustic stimulation from 28 weeks of gestation (Smith, 1994). The observation and assumption that auditory sensation is one of the first to get affected by hypoxia (Arulkumaran, 1992).

It is noteworthy that the original acoustic stimulation test (fetal acoustic stimulation test—FAST) has been renamed as vibroacoustic stimulation test (VAST) because it has been found that vibration element of stimulation is equally if not more important than simple acoustic stimulus (Ingemarsson et al, 1993).

PROCEDURE OF PERFORMING VAST

It is more or less same as that of NST. After fixing the fetal heart transducer on the mother's abdomen, she is asked to turn slightly and lie on her left side. The remote event marker is then given in her hand so that she can indicate her perceived FM by pressing its button. When it is all set, as a first step, 5–10 minutes of nonstress CTG is done. It is noteworthy that if within first 5–10 minutes there occurs spontaneously 2–3 fetal movements with good acceleration of FH—the vibroacoustic stimulus may not be given. If the above has not happened, at the end of this period the fetus is given the stimulus with the help of a vibroacoustic stimulator (see below) by placing it anywhere over the baby's upper half of the body, i.e. somewhat near it's ear but never over it. Eller et al (1992) reported identical FH and FM response whether the stimulator was placed over the vertex or the breech of the fetus.

In a healthy fetus cardiac acceleration occurs almost instantly on giving the stimulus. However, if the 'qualifying acceleration' (see below), fails to occur with one stimulus, it may be repeated at 1–3 minutes intervals for a maximum of three times (see the 'duration of stimulus' below).

Vibroacoustic Stimulator

These are small hand-held battery operated (some have both battery and mains facility) instrument which delivers a mixture of acoustic and vibratory stimulus when switched on (**Fig. 19.1**).

Generally the stimulators are so designed that they generate sound pressure (intensity) between 75 dB to 85 dB at 1 metre in air. The audio frequency of these equipments generally varies between 75 Hz to 85 Hz with harmonics ranging from 20 to 9000 Hz. Here are some names of stimulator that are in use—Corometric model 146, Electronic artificial larynx model 5C, Debdas' vibroacoustic stimulator-mechanical model and electromagnetic model.

Further, it has been found that more fetuses respond to lower frequency acoustic stimulation (e.g. 82 Hz) than higher frequency stimulus (e.g. 1000 or more Hz). This is because abdominal wall and uterine wall attenuate significant degrees of external noises of frequencies higher than 1000 Hz (e.g. 2000 Hz frequency sound delivered at 120 dB level to the fetus may get attenuated to as low as 50 dB level). Hence, it would appear that fetuses do not perceive

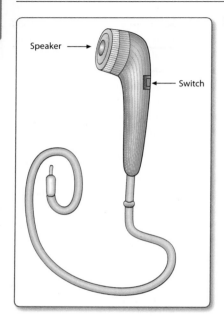

Fig. 19.1 Acoustic stimulator

noises of high frequency (Ingemarsson et al, 1993) and if such quality of stimulus is used VAST may be negative.

Duration of Stimulus

Usually stimulus is given for a period of 1–3 seconds only. More mature the fetus, lesser the duration of stimulus required to elicit 'qualifying response' (see below) because of greater maturity of its cochlear apparatus. Hence for a mature or postdated fetus 1 second stimulus may be enough to elicit the required response. Perhaps based on this, some stimulators are so designed that these deliver their stimulus for a period of maximum three seconds only on one press of the 'ON' button. Some authors have used a maximum of five seconds stimulus in the fetuses who failed to respond to the usual maximum of three seconds but this is not recommended.

Qualifying Response/Acceleration

This means acceleration of FHR by at least 15 bpm, lasting for at least 15 seconds occurring within 15 seconds after the stimulation (Debdas, 1998, William's Obstetrics, 2012).

RESPONSE TO VAST

Basically two types of response may be observed.
- Reactive
- Non-reactive

Reactive VAST (see Figs 13.26 and 13.27)

A VAST can be labeled as 'reactive' -

a. If there occurs two or more FH accelerations of at least 15 bpm, lasting for at least fifteen seconds in a 10 minutes period (Smith et al, 1986) or

b. If there occurs at least one acceleration lasting at least 60 seconds (Arulkumaran, 1992) or

c. If there occurs sustained acceleration (tachycardia) by at least 15 bpm and lasting for at least 3 minutes or more (Arulkumaran, 1992) or

d. If there occurs a series of 2–5 accelerations lasting for 20–60 seconds each (Arias, 1993).

Maternal perception of fetal movement soon after giving the stimulus makes the test even more worthy of labeling as reactive.

It has been observed that most fetuses, whether stimulated during high or low variability phase of FH, continues in high variability after the VAST.

Both FH and FM response of the fetus is greater if stimulation is applied during low FH variability which goes to suggest that in this situation the vibroacoustic stimulation probably serves to wake the fetus up. In fact, VAST is used as a method to exclude fetal sleep in the cases of flat CTG.

Non-Reactive VAST (see Fig. 13.4)

When at least two qualifying accelerations have failed to occur within 10 minutes of giving the stimulus, and undoubtedly so, if it has failed to occur even at the end of 40 minutes after the stimulus—the test should be considered as non-reactive (Smith et al, 1986).

A faster way of knowing the state of fetal reactivity is to repeat the stimulus at 1 minute interval for a maximum of three times (Smith et al, 1986). In author's unit the repeat stimulus is given usually at 3 minutes intervals for the same maximum of three times (see **Fig. 13.4**).

To elaborate on non-reactivity further:

a. Total absence of acceleration is considered ominous

b. Occurrence of deceleration with stimulus is considered serious. In the event of the latter happening, as high as three out of four cases may be found to show fetal distress as evidenced by low scalp pH (Ingemarsson et al, 1993).

Some authors have endeavored to classify the above 'reactive' and 'non-reactive' response into various types (Arulkumaran, 1992 ; Smith, 1994). The following is the classification used in author's unit.

Type I

Prolonged (at least 3 minutes) acceleration by 15 BPM above the baseline.

Type II

Two accelerations by 15 bpm and lasting for at least 15 seconds over 10 minutes period or one such acceleration over the same period but lasting for at least 1 minute.

Type III

a. Transient acceleration lasting for less than 15 seconds (spiky).

b. Suboptimal amplitude of acceleration, i.e. degree of acceleration of less than 15 bpm from baseline.

Type IV

Biphasic response, i.e. an acceleration followed by a deceleration of usually 60 BPM magnitude from the baseline lasting for 60 seconds.

Type V
No acceleration at all.
Type VI
Deceleration following the stimulus.

Of these, Type I and II responses are to be considered as normal response, Type III as suspicious and Type IV, V and VI as abnormal response.

Besides the typical types of responses described above atypical responses to VAST are also seen but no judgement can be given on these.

The fetal response to acoustic stimulation has been assessed by ultrasonography and the following changes in fetal posture and activity have been observed—arching of the back, breathing movement, movement of limbs and movement of eyeballs.

FACTORS THAT MAY INFLUENCE THE RESULT OF VAST

- Thickness of maternal abdominal wall (obesity).
- The amount of amnioitic fluid.
- Pressure exerted by the examiner in holding the stimulator against the abdomen.
- Intensity (dB) of the stimulation.
- The state of the battery of the stimulator—weak battery will give weak stimulation and hence may fail to stimulate the fetus.

However, influence of these factors have been estimated to be very small since only 2 percent NSTs are non-reactive following VAST.

HABITUATION (TO VAST)

Habituation to VAST is generally defined as failure of the fetus to respond to repetitive application of the stimulus *after an initial qualifying response*. According to Smith et al (1991) the mean number of stimulus required for habituation is about five and it can range from one to ten.

It has been suggested that habituation represent a basic example of learning and hence it probably requires an intact central nervous system (Smith, 1994).

It has been found that infants who fail to habituate are more likely to be small for date, have meconium stained liquor or major nervous system malformation like microcephaly, anencephaly, etc. They also have been reported to have higher incidence of cesarean section for fetal distress, low Apgar and gross placental anomaly like infarction and abruption (Smith et al, 1991; Smith, 1994).

However, usefulness of habituation as a clinical tool is not established.

VAST—AN EIGHT PARAMETER TEST

VAST directly or indirectly elicits and thereby tests the following fetal systems or functions:
- Functional state of CNS
- Reflex CVS response to CNS stimulation
- Startle response
- Motor response (flexion-extension type of limb movement)
- Ability of integration (Intact somatomotor sensory pathway)
- Auditory acuity
- Fetal behavior
- Fetal learning ability (see habituation).

VAST AND PRE-TERM FETUS

In pregnancies of duration less than 36 weeks VAST gives unusual FHR pattern which are difficult to interpret and hence this test is not very useful in these cases (Smith, 1994).

Predictive Value of Vast for Antenatal Fetal Surveillance

As an antenatal test for fetal well-being—the overall fetal death rate following a reactive VAST has been reported to be as low as 1.9 per 1000 (Smith, 1994). Using VAST and amniotic fluid volume assessment Clark et al (1989) reported no unexpected fetal death amongst 5973 tests.

Read and Miller (1977) reported that VAST is as reliable test of antenatal fetal well-being as the CST—a test which is considered as a very sensitive test of fetal well-being (though very cumbersome, time consuming and slightly risky).

More recently, bi-weekly VAST with AFI has been reported to be an excellent test of fetal well being with False negative result of 0.8% and false positive result of 1.5% (William's Obstetrics, 2012)

PLACE OF VAST FOR INTRAPARTUM FETAL MONITORING

Vibroacoustic stimulation test can be used in labor for the following two purposes :
- As an 'Admission test'
- As an alternative to FBS.

Vast as an 'Admission Test'

For this, on admission in labor, after 10 minutes of conventional NST, the fetus is given an acoustic stimulation and the consequent FHR changes noted and interpreted.

The VAST offers a better predictive value as an 'admission test' than the conventional NST alone.

Vast as an Alternative to FBS

FBS is one of the recommended method of double checking abnormal CTG tracing by measuring the pH value of fetal blood and noting whether it was in acidosis range or otherwise. This is because it has been found that if the fetus has not gone into the stage of metabolic acidosis, which is an indicator occurrence of more severe degree of hypoxia, i.e. the tissue hypoxia, it is very unlikely to suffer brain damage even in presence of abnormal CTG and hence one can avoid premature interference, i.e. emergency operative delivery in these cases.

However, in spite of this solid reason and the reported incidence of 50 percent false positivity of conventional NST, this facility and expertise for doing FBS is not available in most centres using CTG monitoring even in developed countries, even over 30 years after its introduction. It has been reported that less than half the units in UK who use CTG to monitor labor has got this facility and there are many sound reasons (outside the purview of the present topic) for not adopting FBS as a routine second line method.

Certainly, in comparison to FBS and pH, VAST is an ultra simple, non-invasive, instant, easily repeatable, low skilled and reasonably effective method. Here are some evidence on the reliability of the method—

a. It has been found that majority of non-acidotic fetuses respond to VAST by acceleration even in presence of abnormal CTG tracing (Arulkumaran, 1992).

b. No fetus who responds to VAST by the qualifying degree of acceleration is found to have acidotic pH (Smith, 1994). This has been found to be true even in the cases of suspicious and ominous trace.

However, two exceptions to the above generalisation are note-worthy:

Not all, only 50 percent of those with abnormal NST trace who fail to respond to VAST show acidic pH. So, it would appear that VAST can avoid the necessity of FBS in at least 50 percent cases and thereby reduce the interference rate in the same proportion in the presence of abnormal NST (Arulkumaran, 1992, William's Obstetrics, 2012).

Besides, it has been shown that with respiratory acidosis, which is considered as an evidence of mild hypoxia, reactive VAST is possible but with metabolic acidosis, as a general rule, VAST gives non-reactive response.

USES AND ADVANTAGES OF VAST AS A METHOD FOR FETAL SURVEILLANCE

1. It reduces the 'duration' of non-stress CTG monitoring by 50 percent which is of benefit both for the mother (less discomfort) and also for the medical care provider, e.g. employer of the patient, Government health department, etc. (reduces cost). This benefit is additive—more the monitoring load, greater is the saving of man and machine time. To it also must be added the saving of the expensive paper that is used for tracing.

2. It reduces the 'incidence' of non-reactive NST by 50 percent (Smith et al, 1986).

3. It directly or indirectly tests eight functions or systems of the fetus as already mentioned.

4. VAST is a good screening test for the oxygen status of the fetus on admission in labour—the so-called 'Admission Test'.

5. VAST can also serve as an alternative to 'fetal blood sampling' in labor and thereby reduces the necessity of this invasive procedure. Reactive VAST is more reliable evidence of absence of hypoxia and Acidosis in presence of Variable Deceleration in CTG than when Late Deceleration is present (Lin et al, 2001).

6. It is useful in better visualisation of fetal anatomy specially during anomaly scan because 95 percent fetus change their position after vibroacoustic stimulation. This often shifts fetus from unfavourable position to a favourable one for critical scanning.

7. It is an extremely useful method for excluding fetal sleep in the cases showing prolonged low FH variability on NST.

8. It's operation is very simple—can be done by a nurse.

9. It is noninvasive.

10. It is easily repeatable.

11. VAST plus AFI constitute the modified biophysical profile testing which takes only 10 minutes to perform and which is now considered as a superb method of antepartum fetal surveillance (Clark et al, 1989, William's Obstetrics, 2012).

COMPARABILITY OF VAST WITH OTHER INTRAPARTUM FETAL SURVEILLANCE TESTS

A meta-analysis done of reports on intrapartum fetal stimulation tests published between 1966 to 2000 found that VAST is as reliable test of fetal wellbeing as – scalp puncture for doing FBS, pinch of the scalp with Allis tissue forceps and scalp stimulation test (Skupski et al, 2002).

SAFETY OF VAST

No damage to the auditory acuity has been demonstrated in babies exposed to VAST during the third trimester on screening the newborn at 1 to 2 days of age and again at 4 years of age (Arulkumaran and Montan, 1991).

VAST has not been found to endanger neurological development in exposed infants (Smith, 1994).

No significant increase in adrenaline or nonadrenaline concentrations was found in cord blood after VAST—the chemicals which may be harmful for the fetus (Arulkumaran and Montan, 1991).

VAST has been blamed to force a growth restricted fetus to spend more energy when it is trying to conserve it by remaining inactive. In these cases it is better to do biophysical profile without VAST and Doppler velocimetry than VAST.

FURTHER READING

1. American College of Obstetrics & Gynecology (ACOG): Antepartum Fetal Surveillance, Practice Bulletein No. 9, 2007.
2. Arias F. Practical Guide to High Risk Pregnancy and Delivery (2nd edn), St Louis: Mosby. 1993;3–20:301–18,413–29.
3. Arulkumaran S. In: Ratnam SS, Bhasker Rao K, Arulkumaran S (Eds). Obstetrics and Gynaecology for Postgraduates. Hyderabad: Orient Longman, 1992;115–26.
4. Arulkumaran S, Montan S. Singapore Journal of Obstetrics and Gynaecology 1991;22(2):35–39.

5. Clark SL, Sabey P, Jolley K. Nonstress testing with acoustic stimulation and amniotic fluid volume assessment: 5973 tests without unexpected fetal death. Am J Obstet Gynaecol 1989;160:694.

6. Cunningham FG, Gant NF, Leveno KJ. William's Obstetrics (21st edn), New York: McGraw-Hill, 2001;347:1103–05.

7. Debdas AK. Practical Cardiotocography (1st edn), Delhi: Jaypee Brothers 1998;143–52:166–8.

8. Devoe LD: Antenatal fetal Assessment: Multifetal gestation—an overview, Semin Perinatology, 2008 32:281.

9. Eller PD, Robinson LJ, Newman RB. Am J Obstet Gynaecol 1992;167:1137–9.

10. Hykin J, More R, Duncan K, et al. Fetal brain activity demonstrated by functional magnetic resonance imaging. Lancet 1989;354:645.

11. Ingemarsson I, Ingemarsson V, Spencer JAD. Fetal Heart Rate Monitoring—A Practical Guide. Oxford: Oxford University Press, 1993;283–5.

12. Lin CC, Vassallo B, Mittendrof R : Is Intrapartum Vibroacoustic stimulation an effective predictor of fetal acidosis, J Perinat Med 2001;29:506.

13. Read JA, Miller FC. Am J Obstet Gynaecol 1977;129:512.

14. Skupski DW, Rosenburg CR: Intrapartum fetal stimulation tests—a meta-analysis, Eglinton GS, Obstet Gynecol, 2002;99:129.

15. Smith CV, Phelan JP, Plat LW, et al. Am J Obstet Gynaecol 1986;155:131–4.

16. Smith CV, Davis SN, Rayburn WF, Nelson RM. Am J Perinatology 1991;8:(6):380–82.

17. Smith CV. Vibroacoustic stimulation for risk assessment: In Clinics in Perinatology 1994;21:797–808.

18. William's Obstetrics: 23rd edition, Edited by Cunningham FG, Leveno KJ, Bloom SL, Hauth JC, Rouse DJ and Spong CY, Intrapartum Assessment, Mc Graw Hill, New York, 2010;340, 342, 427.

Computer Analysis of CTG Trace

THE NEED

Certainly since late sixties Cardiotocography (CTG) has become an integral part of obstetric practice though originally introduced in the late fifties. But despite this long years of use, the interpretation of tracing features still varies from doctor to doctor. The main reason for this has been found to be the fact that the analysis is done *visually*. For example, Keith et al (1995) asked each of 17 experts to review 50 tracings on two occasions, at least one month apart. About 20 percent changed their own interpretation, and approximately 25 percent did not agree with the interpretation of their colleagues.

THE AIM

Computer analysis of fetal heart rate (FHR) aims to do the following:
- Remove the drawback of subjective visual analysis
- Incorporate hard mathematical objectivity to the analysis
- Spell out precisely—what is normal and what is abnormal?

THE BASIS

This revolutionary technique has been developed in the early eighties by Professor GS Dawes and Professor C Redman of UK by computer analysis of 40,000 antenatal CTG tracings. Based on it, they have developed an algorithm which now analyses the test cases. The new generation of CTG machines with computer analysis software is now widely available.

Software Specification

The machine takes the CTG and then analyses it on the following criteria (Sonicaid product description, Oxford Instruments, UK, Publication No. 8902 – 8502 and Laybourn and Mander, 2000):

Accelerations

The following two definitions are used to evaluate acceleration:

a. A rise in FHR from the baseline of more than 10 bpm and lasting longer than fifteen15 seconds.

b. A rise in FHR from the baseline of more than 15 bpm and lasting longer than 15 seconds.

Although these are not considered to be a good enough predictor of normality they are included in the analysis as they are the traditional feature identified visually.

Decelerations

The software counts the number of decelerations that occurred and also lists those with 50 or more lost beats on the report.

It is noteworthy here that in this approach deceleration is counted in terms of 'lost beats' (e.g. if the graph drops by 20 bpm below baseline and stays there for 2 minutes, the number of heart beat 'lost' would be $20 \times 2 = 40$).

Long-term Variation

This is found out by 'individually' analysing each minute's tracing for the minimum and the maximum FHR and the difference between the two is then worked out. These figures are then averaged.

Here the evaluation is done not in terms of BPM but in terms of 'pulse interval difference' measured in msec. The pulse interval difference means the time interval between consecutive beats.

Episode of High (and Low) Variation

An episode of high variation is a section of the trace where 5 out of 6 consecutive minutes have a variation which is above the threshold for higher limit of variation. Similarly, for low variation, limit of lower threshold is taken.

The record is considered to be abnormal if there is no episode of high variation.

Basal Heart Rate

This is taken to be the average FHR during episodes of low variation.

Short-term Variability

This is found out by averaging FHR for every epoch of 3.75 seconds. Again here FHR is calculated not as BPM but as pulse interval difference as mentioned above.

The Mother's Assessment of Fetal Movement

This is expressed as *movement per hour*. Mother is given a remote event marker in her hand. She is advised to press its button as and when she feels a definite fetal movement which is automatically noted (printed) on the tracing paper.

Uterine Contraction

A contraction is recorded if the external uterine pressure rises more than 16 percent for 30 seconds or more.

Signal Loss

This is calculated in percentage and an alarm sounds if it exceeds 30 percent in any 10 minutes period.

Dawes-Redman Criteria of Normalcy

For the system 8002 machine of sonicaid—this has been derived from the analysis of over 48,000 records. This software provides the rules for determining whether the tracing of a patient is *normal or abnormal*.

1. There must be an episode of high variation which should be above the 1st centile for gestational age.
   Note: High variation is a sign of normality.
2. The mean variation during all episodes of high variation must be greater than 32 msecs.
3. The overall variation must be greater than 22 msecs.
4. The short term variation must be greater than 3 msecs. Recently, greater emphasis is being placed on the measurement of short-term variation (STV) rather than long-term variation. Whereas STV value of 4+ is associated with 0 percent incidence of acidaemia and intrauterine death, value less than 2.5 is associated with 72 percent of these anomalies (Street et al, 1991; Laybourn and Mander, 2000).
5. There must be no decelerations of more than 20 lost beats or any deceleration (regardless of size) at the end of the record.
6. There should be no evidence of Sinusoidal heart rhythm.
7. The basal heart rate must be between 116 and 160 bpm.
8. There must be at least one fetal movement sensed by the mother.

Operation

After fixing the CTG machine (system 8002, Sonicaid) on the patient, it should be run continuously for 10 minutes to fit a 'baseline' from the initial analysis of this 10 minutes data. After that, analysis is automatically performed every 2 minutes, and the result updated (see **Fig. 20.1** showing a typical auto analysed report).

Out of eight parameters of analysis six can be viewed on the LCD located on the front panel of the machine. The printer gives the print out as and when required.

The computerised machine has a 6 hour memory capability.

The base unit of the machine can be used in the patient's home at a remote site and the emerging CTG data can be sent by telephone to a central base station (telemetry).

These type of machines usually also has language option for the following languages—English, German, French, Italian and Spanish.

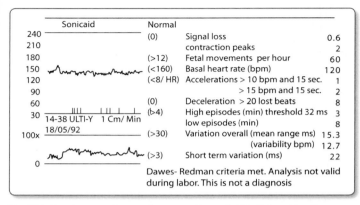

Sonicaid	Normal		
	(0)	Signal loss	0.6
		contraction peaks	2
	(>12)	Fetal movements per hour	60
	(<160)	Basal heart rate (bpm)	120
	(<8/ HR)	Accelerations > 10 bpm and 15 sec.	1
		> 15 bpm and 15 sec.	2
	(0)	Deceleration > 20 lost beats	8
14-38 ULTI-Y 1 Cm/ Min	(b>4)	High episodes (min) threshold 32 ms	3
18/05/92		low episodes (min)	8
	(>30)	Variation overall (mean range ms)	15.3
		(variability bpm)	12.7
	(>3)	Short term variation (ms)	22

Dawes- Redman criteria met. Analysis not valid during labor. This is not a diagnosis

Fig. 20.1 Showing a sample report from sonicaid team S-8000 CTG machine. Note the analysis on the right hand side of the chart (with permission from Dr Terry Martin, Business Director, Sonicaid Products)

Special Advantages of the Autoanalysing CTG Machines

- It turns a subjective visual assessment into an objective test.
- It can evaluate very subtle changes in the CTG which is impossible by a human eye.
- It is nonoperator dependent.
- It reduces the monitoring time.
- It is more reliable.
- As opposed to conventional CTG, which is good only for predicting healthy fetus, Computer analysed CTG method has been reported to be good both for predicting healthy fetus and also sick fetus (Laybourne and Mander, 2000).
- There are reports that there has been reduction in cesarean section rate and also of fetal mortality and morbidity rate by its use in comparison to the use of conventional CTG.

- Since the data is stored electronically, it enables detailed research and audit to be undertaken. Hence, it provides a good basis for evidence based medicine.

Scope

The system has been developed for the management of high-risk pregnancy during the antenatal period from 26 weeks onwards. Presently, it is not suitable for the intrapartum period (Sonicaid product description).

Future of Computerisation of CTG Tracing and Reporting

The focus of research on this technique is now on its applicability for intrapartum traces. Two new software is under trial for this namely—'Matching pursuit' and 'Detranded analysis'. However, the prediction of computer analysis and umbilical artery acidosis have not been found to correlate well. According to a recent report, computer analysis of 'low-low frequency' parameter appear to recognise the occurrence of fetal acidosis with greater sensitivity and specificity (Agarwal et al, 2003; Salamalekis et al, 2006).

FURTHER READING

1. Agarwal SK, Doucette F, Gratton R, et al Intrapartum computerised fetal heart rate parameters and Metabolic Acidosis at birth, Obstet Gynecol: 2003;102:731–8

2. Edwin C and Arulkumaran S: Electronic Fetal Heart Monitoring in current & future practice, The Journal of O & G of India, 2008; 58: 121–30.

3. Keith RDF, Beckley S, Garibaldi JM, et al. Brist J Obstet Gynaecol, 1995;102:688.

4. Laybourn M, Mander AM. Progress in Obstetrics and Gynaecology. Studd J 2000;14:188–201.

5. Salamalekis E, Hintipas E, Salloum I, et al. Computerised analysis of fetal heart rate variability using the matching pursuit technique as an indicator of fetal hypoxia in labor, J Matern Fetal Neonatol Med, 19: 2006;165–9.

6. Sonicaid TEAM Fetal monitor-user's guide: Publication No. 8909-8500, Issue -2, Kimber Road, Oxford, UK, 45–73, 99–111, 143–4.

7. Sonicaid TEAM S-8000 printer - Product description, Publication No. 8902 -8502, Oxford Instruments, Oxford, UK.

8. Street P, Dawes GS, Moulden M, Redman CWG. Am J Obstet Gynecol 1991;165:515–23.

CTG Cum Fetal ECG—An Approach Towards Precision

BASIS

Just as in myocardial infarction/ischemia in adult, presence of abnormal ST wave in F-ECG also denotes fetal myocardial ischemia/acidosis and its absence oxygenated state.

SCOPE

Fetal surveillance during labor constitutes a challenge in information management. To give birth is a natural process for women but for the child it may constitute a threat for intact survival and ominous changes may appear within minutes.

Misinterpretation of the CTG not only causes an increase in unnecessary intervention but it is also implicated in a large proportion of patients with birth asphyxia and avoidable perinatal morbidity. Since physiologically, a multitude of factors influence FH Rate in the term fetus we really cannot expect that there would be distinct FHR features in CTG traces that would be specific enough to discriminate between *different levels of hypoxia* though CTG, which is a *rate based technology*, certainly provides very valid information about fetal reactiveness. May be that is why, in many cases, experts cannot agree on the significance of CTG changes and also whether the hypoxic brain injury occurred before or during labor or whether it was preventable by an emergency delivery.

It is also recognised that although many fetuses face periods of relative oxygen deficiency during labor, very few suffer long-term damage as a result. Indeed, even the consequences of a severe lack of oxygen will vary from one fetus to another.

Most importantly, as high as 50% of all those fetuses who show grossly abnormal CTG do not show evidence of occurrence of metabolic acidosis – the final marker of tissue hypoxia.

Don't all these call for an easy instant adjunct to CTG which should be able to assess -

- **the tissue hypoxia**
- **of a very vital organ-the fetal heart**
- **'side by side' with CTG procedure**
- **by the same machine**
- **in the same sitting.**

Incorporation of F-ECG with CTG is an endeavor towards this end.

Pathophysiological Basis of Using F-ECG (Rosen, 2003)

Biophysics

This has been shown schematically in **Figure 21.1**. The waveform marked P corresponds to the contraction of the atrium and the complex Q,R,S immediate following this—the contraction of the ventricles. The generation of these waveforms are passive events and thus very stable and easily detected which makes it well suited for fetal heart rate recording. The *ST waveform*, which depicts the vital, physiologically active component of heart function and which gives maximum information of the *state of cardiac oxygenation*, on the other hand, are more easily affected by signal noise, mode of ECG recording, etc. However, recently, Neoventa Medical AB has developed technique of avoiding these and produce an excellent F-ECG.

Biochemistry

The ST segment and T wave relate to the repolarisation of myocardial cells in preparation for the next contraction. This repolarisation process is energy consuming. An *increase in T wave height*, quantified by the ratio between T and QRS amplitudes, the T/QRS ratio, occurs when the energy balance within the myocardial cells threatens to become negative. A negative energy balance means a situation when the amount of oxygen supplied to the cells no longer cover the energy required for metabolic activity. During hypoxia this balance becomes negative and the cells produce energy by the beta adrenoceptor mediated anaerobic breakdown of glycogen reserves. The ability of these cells to produce energy in this manner and thereby maintain myocardial function is a vital compensatory defense mechanism. This process not only produces lactic acid but also potassium ions (K^+) which affects myocardial cell membrane potential and cause a rise of the ST waveform. Thus, the rise in T wave amplitude and increase in T/QRS ratio reflects the rate of myocardial glycogenolysis and the utilisation of a key fetal defence to hypoxia.

Note

Besides hypoxemia, these ST changes can also occur as a result of general surge of stress hormones (adrenaline) occurring in response to the squeezing and squashing of labor. This will stimulate the heart to increase its pumping activity but at the same time induce glycogenolysis and high T waves. This general arousal is part of normal labor and in these cases the healthy fetus will display a reactive CTG ensuring normality.

Understanding ST Events (Rosen, 2003)

Basically the inference about fetal hypoxia is drawn on the following two ST events both of which are ominous (**Fig. 21.1**):

- *Increase of T height* – Evidence of early hypoxia (see above)
- *T wave depression* – Evidence of late hypoxia (see below)

ST depression with negative T waves has been observed during hypoxia experiments in experimentally growth retarded guinea pigs. They reflect a myocardium that is not able or had not had the time to mobilise its defence to hypoxemia. The result is a decrease in myocardial activity and a risk of cardiovascular failure.

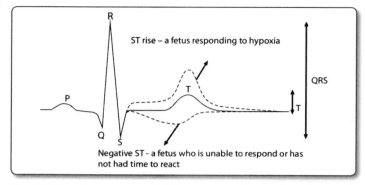

Fig. 21.1 Schematic presentation of F-ECG showing normal T wave (the solid lined middle trace) and elevated and depressed T waves—the two broken lined traces. Both elevated and depressed T waves are evidences of fetal hypoxia. Elevation signifies that the fetus is responding to hypoxia by using its reserves whereas depression signifies it is unable to respond or has not had time to respond. Notice two arrows on the right hand side showing the relative height of QRS (R) and T – the T/QRS ratio

The physiology behind biphasic ST events is related to the mechanical performance of the myocardium and the relationship between the inner (endocardium) and outer (epicardium) layers of the walls of the ventricles in particular. As we know, biphasic ST illustrates an imbalance between these two layers, the reason being that the perfusion pressure of the endocardium is always lower while the mechanical strain is always greater. This means that unless the myocardium is generally activated (beta receptor activation and enhanced Frank-Starling relationship, i.e. the ability of the myocardium to respond to volume load), any decrease in performance will cause biphasic ST. Thus, not only hypoxia *per se* may cause biphasic ST as a sign of maladaptation, but also basically all factors substantially altering the balance within the myocardial wall may institute these events.

Clinical Examples of Intracardiac Imbalance

- **Prematurity** with less contractile elements making the heart less capable of responding to shifts in volume load and decreased ability to respond with glycogenolysis.

- **Infections** ranging from general septicemia to non-specific inflammatory reactions can affect by altering membrane–pumping mechanisms and reducing myocardial performance.
- **Increase demand on the cardiovascular system** as may be seen with an *increase in temperature* or simply by a *marked tachycardia* by itself. These situations may not be specific enough to cause an alarm reaction but a slight ST depression may just inform that the myocardium is required to enhance its pumping performance somewhat beyond its optimum.
- **Fetal Myocardial dystrophy.** An idiopathic condition of poor performance in utero, recovering spontaneously after birth.
- **Cardiac malformations.**
- **Long-term stress** causing inability of the myocardium to adapt to emerging hypoxia
- In the **acute hypoxic phase**, before adrenaline activation of beta adrenoceptors.

Basically, biphasic ST is the pattern to be expected whenever the myocardium is exposed to factors that may decrease its ability to respond.

Probably the most clinically important aspect of display of **biphasic ST is**—once it has been flagged it means a **situation of potentially reduced myocardial performance** has been identified. But at this stage "classical" signs of fetal reactions to an emerging hypoxia is not to be expected, i.e. metabolic acidosis, etc. However, with further progress of labour and during 2nd stage in particular, these fetuses will suffer.

Technical Requirement for Doing Fetal ECG

It is simply an extension of 'internal' method of CTG monitoring and as usual needs placement of an electrode on fetal scalp or buttock. The only additional requirment is STAN (S-T analyser) software fed into the CTG machine for analysis and interpretation of the emerging ECG.

Clinical Results

According to earlier reports, this system have shown reduction of both operative delivery for fetal distress and also the incidence of umbilical artery metabolic acidosis (Amer-Wahlin et al, 2001; Westgate et al, 1993) though more recent study by Doria et al in 2007 did not find any such difference.

According to Cochrane database involving the analysis of 8872 cases, the conclusion was—STAN is perhaps useful in preventing fetal acidosis and neonatal encephalopathy when standard FHR monitoring suggested abnormal pattern (Neilson, 2006). Randomised control on the use of this technique has not been conducted yet in USA (William's obstetrics, 2010).

Alternatives to F-ECG

Fetal Blood Sampling (FBS) and pH Estimation

Fetal blood sampling can be used along with CTG monitoring to assess fetal acid-base status during labor and can reduce operative intervention but it requires additional expertise, is time consuming, gives only intermittent information and is not therefore widely used.

CTG Plus Pulse Oximetry

The snag here is, level of oxygen in blood may not always reflect the state of oxygen utilization by the vital, high oxygen priority organs like heart and brain because this depends on many other local and general factors. In this context, assessment of impact of hypoxemia 'on the function' of these organs may be a better proposition as can be done, e.g. F-ECG.

Technical Advantages of F-ECG

1. Its simplicity—Can be obtained just by the flick of a switch at any time from any patient who is on internal CTG monitoring because in this technique the FHR is actually derived from F-ECG only. So, the fetal electrode is already in situ. All that is needed is incorporation of STAN (ST Analyser) software. No additional instrumentation or handling of the patient is required.
2. Very low skill requirement—in comparison to FBS and Pulse oxymetry.

3. Does direct assessment of the impact of hypoxia on a high priority vital organ, namely heart—depicts the ability of the heart to cope with the total stress.

FURTHER READING

1. Amer-Wåhlin I, Hellsten C, Norén H, Hagberg H, Herbst A, Kjellmer I, et al. Intrapartum Fetal Monitoring: Cardiotocography versus Cardiotocography plus ST Analysis of the Fetal ECG. A Swedish Randomized Controlled Trial. Lancet, 2001;358:534–8.

2. Amer-Wåhlin I, Arulkumaran S, Hagberg H, et al. Fetal Electrocardiogram: ST wave form analysis in intrapartum surveillance, BJOG, 2007;114:1191.

3. Doria V, Papageorghiou AT, et al. Review of the first 1502 cases of ECG-ST wave form analysis during labor in a teaching hospital, BJOG:2007;114:1202.

4. Neilson JP et al. Fetal Electrocardiogram (ECG) for fetal monitoring during labor, Cochrane Database System Review 3: CD 000116 l, 2006.

5. Rosen KG, Amer-Wåhlin I, Luzietti R, et al. Fetal ECG wave form analysis; Best Pract Res Clin Obstet Gynecol: 2004;13: 485–514

6. Rosen KG. In Practical Obstetrics, Edited by Debdas AK, Jaypee, New Delhi, 2003;1:163–72.

7. Westgate J, Harris M, Curnow JSH, Greene KR. Plymouth randomised trial of cardiotocogram only versus ST waveform plus cardiotocogram for intrapartum monitoring: 2,400 cases. Am J Obstet Gynaecol, 1993;169:1151–60.

8. William's Obstetrics: 23rd edition, Edited by Cunningham FG, Leveno KJ, Bloom SL, Hauth JC, Rouse DJ and Spong CY, Intrapartum Assessment, Mc Graw Hill, New York, 2010;428–9.

Non-reassuring CTG Trace

Dellinger et al (2000) conducted a study of 'just the tracing characters' and found almost a third of the tracings examined were of the so-called 'intermediate type' which means that these were neither absolutely normal nor overtly abnormal. This type of tracings were also assessed at the fetal monitoring workshop conducted by NICHD (National Institute of Child Health and Human Development) in 1997 where also there emerged no consensus on these. Hence is the genesis of the term 'non-reassuring trace'.

But this is not simply a matter of fixing a terminology, there are far more serious problems to it because it has been reported that 70% of all liability claims related to brain damage are based on abnormality of Fetal Heart Rate tracing of CTG (Cardiotocography). So, how to fix gravity on these intermediate or not so abnormal kind of trace.

What is a Non-reassuring Trace

Any CTG trace which is not absolutely normal on all the standard parameters of assessment is a non-reassuring trace. Looking at it from another angle this term is nothing but an all encompassing logical new name for equivocal CTG trace. Let us analyse the logic for this rephrasing.

While most obstetricians all these years have been taking all such off mark traces *as signs of fetal distress* and had been acting upon these accordingly, it is quite a common experience that such apprehensive assumption does not prove to be correct in very significant number of cases. However, based on the above befooling experience (often first hand) one cannot afford to take the risk of ignoring such traces because, as already mentioned, it may well be a sign of real fetal hypoxia in some cases and in such cases one may be sued for causing brain damage if not for the occurrence of stillbirth.

So, when an obstetrician faces any such trace, he or she sinks into a state of disquieting indecision as Cunningham et al (2001) have very aptly put it—'in this situation, obstetricians essentially experience surges of both confidence and doubt', i.e. he or she is not re-assured either way as to whether it is a true sign of fetal distress or it is a variant of normal fetal heart response. Based on the above if one looks at it critically, it would appear that what really the non-reassuring traces cause is – it induces *'Obstetrician's distress'*.

To summarise it all in one line, any tracing which is not absolutely normal/high class *from all angles* is a 'non-reassuring' trace.

The Possible Scientific Explanations for the Occurrence of Non-reassuring Traces

1. Since FHR pattern results from complex interactions of intrinsic multifactorial control mechanisms like – parasympathetic and sympathetic surges, the state of myocardial conduction pathways, as well as the inherent cardiac reflex arcs – small changes in fetal homeostasis, therefore are reflected in altered FHR patterns and may cause confusion.
2. CTG assesses the fetal 'physiological response' rather than patho-logical response Cunningham et al 2001 and hence cannot be a very efficient parameter for assessing pathological events.
3. CTG, technically, is a simply 'rate' based method, i.e. based only on the analysis 'rate' (of fetal heart)– a parameter which inherently is a very labile and dynamic system and hence can become abnormal and normal again within a very short time, even for flimsy reasons.

Inter-observer Variability and the Problem of Labeling a Tracing as Reassuring or Non-reassuring

The above variability in interpretation arises because the tracings are assessed by simple visual estimation which necessarily suffer from the drawback of subjectivity, and it is not only the inter-observer even the intra-observer variability in interpretation does occur due to the same reason. This has been amply demonstrated by Keith et al [1995] who asked each of the 17 experts to review 50 tracings on two occasions at least one month apart and this is what they found : about 20% changed their own interpretation and approximately 25% did not agree with the interpretation of their colleagues.

Some Common Practical Examples of Non-reassuring trace and the Under Current it Generates

- Not all, only one or two features of the tracing are abnormal-causing mental disturbance to the obstetrician.
- A feature is abnormal but for duration shorter than the accepted definition, for example, for the abnormality of baseline FHR it should be present for a minimum period of 10 minutes but even 5 minutes **may be unbearable** for the obstetrician specially if it is recurrent or the rate is too low – in two figures, i.e. below 100/minute. Then, of course, in the back yard of mind flashes the sight of the hanging sword of law suit. According to FIGO (1987)–there must be three or more late deceleration following 'consecutive' contractions for a diagnosis of late deceleration to be made. Obstetricians need to be *tensely patient*! In the above two examples, lack of thorough knowledge and experience about CTG is the main underlying cause of worry.
- The tracing is intermittently abnormal with normal pattern in between – *disturbing!*
- Atypical tracing – a tracing that cannot be fitted into any classically abnormal type – *disturbing* !

Some Possible 'Non-hypoxic Causes' of Non-reassuring CTG Trace

These have been discussed in detail in Chapter 12–'CTG Interpretation–Theoretical Considerations', in summary, this is what these are:

- Contact loss – Loss of contact or improper contact of the abdominal FH transducer or fetal electrode can cause big dips or bizzare tracing.

- Maternal sedation – This must be excluded in all cases of flat CTG trace.
- Maternal tachycardia – Can cause fetal tachycardia.
- Maternal pyrexia – Can cause fetal tachycardia.
- Fetal sleep—This is a common cause of flat CTG trace (see Chapter 18)
- Epidural analgesia – All type of FHR pattern abnormality have been reported with this form of analgesia (see Chapter 24).

These factors must be excluded as the first step in the management of non-reassuring trace.

MANAGEMENT OF NON-REASSURING CTG TRACE

There are two aspects of management:
I. Management of the trace
II. Management of the case

Management of the Trace

This is to be done in order to confirm or refute whether the trace in question constitute a sign of fetal distress or not and this entails the following :

a. Check the contact of the FH transducer, apply some more aquasonic gel. During PV, check the attachment of scalp electrode.
b. Exclude or manage, if present, the non-hypoxic causes of the non-reassuring trace (see below).
c. Continue tracing in the mean time to see what turn it takes
d. Double-check the state of fetal oxygenation by an additional test (see Chapter 23 – 'Beyond CTG').

Management of the Case

This entails the following:
a. Start oxygen inhalation.
b. Reassess the whole case clinically

This is necessary in order to be able to take decision on the totality of the situation.

- Whether it is a case of bad obstetric history
- Whether she is elderly and/or has history of infertility
- What is the state of maturity of the fetus
- Whether she is hypertensive or has any other medical disorder.
- What is the situation about her ***Inducibility and deliverability***. To this end a vaginal examination should be done specially to assess the cervix. In an intranatal case—presentation, position, station, pelvis and colour of liquor are also to be checked. For the last parameter, amniotony have to be done if the membranes are intact.

c. *Making arrangement for immediate delivery if need be* This involves alerting operation theatre, anesthetist, pediatrician and drawing and sending patient's blood for crossmatching.

How to exclude/manage (if present) the non-hypoxic causes of non-reassuring trace.

- Check if mother had any CNS depressant drug.
- Check fetal maturity—baseline tachycardia, reduced baseline variability, poor or absent fetal movement acceleration are sometimes normally exhibited by the fetuses under 34 weeks of gestation.
- Change the position of the mother specially if she was lying supine – to left lateral position. If she was already on lateral decubitus – turn her to lie on the other side. Venacaval compression and positional cord compression specially where liquor volume is less get corrected by doing this.
- Check maternal pulse (see above).
- Check maternal temperature (see above).
- Check maternal BP—if hypotensive – tracing abnormality is possible, e.g. as in a case of epidural.
- Discontinue oxytocin if she has been on it.
- Start intravenous fluids if the mother is hypotensive or dehydrated.

Conclusion

In CTG monitoring non-reassuring trace is a fact of life. However, with increasing experience and knowledge of the user its incidence decreases. A number of simple observations and precautions as mentioned above can reduce the obstetrician's distress that it induces.

FURTHER READING

1. Cunningham FG, Gant NF, Leveno KJ et al: Williams Obstetrics, 21st ed, McGraw-Hill, New York, 2001;346-54:1100–08.
2. Dellinger EH, Boehm FH, Crane MM: Electronic fetal heart rate monitoring: Early neonatal outcomes associated with normal rate, fetal stress and fetal distress. Am J Obstet Gynaecol, 2000;182:214.
3. FIGO "Guidelines for the use of fetal monitoring". Int J Obstet Gynecol, 1987;25:159–67.
4. Keith RDF, Backley S, Garibaldi JM et al: Brit J Obstet Gynaecol 1995;102:688.
5. NICE (National Institute for Clinical Excellance) Guideline: The use of Electronic fetal monitoring: the use and interpretation of Cardiotocography in Intrapartum Fetal Surveillance, 2001, London
6. NICE (National Institute for Clinical Excellance) Guideline :The Clinical Guideline No. 70, Induction of labour, RCOG press, 2008, London
7. NICE (National Institute for Clinical Excellance) Guideline :The Clinical Guideline No. 55, Induction of labour, RCOG press, September 2007, London
8. Symonds EM: Fetal monitoring : Medical and implications for the practitioner, Current Opinion Obstet Gynaecol 1994;6:430.
9. William's Obstetrics: 23rd Edition, Edited by Cunningham FG, Leveno KJ, Bloom SL, Hauth JC, Rouse DJ and Spong CY, Intrapartum Assessment, Mc Graw Hill, New York, 2010;410–43

Beyond CTG

Need to Look Beyond

Here is to quote very disturbing and most quoted studies:

- "Even with the worst pattern of tracing only 50 to 60 percent of fetuses were found to be Acidotic" (Beard, 1971; Konje and Taylor, 1998).
- One third (1/3) of all CTG tracings are found to be of "intermediate" type, i.e. they are –
  - Neither overtly Pathological
  - Nor clearly NORMAL

and these were classed as – "NON-REASSURING" trace !!!

(*NICD-Consensus development workshop, 1997; Dellinger et al, 2000*).

So, undoubtedly the Obstetric speciality needs to look beyond CTG.

Technical Weakness of CTG as a Test of Fetal Well Being

Looking at it critically, the technology CTG has been designed to monitor a physiological response and not a pathological process. It simply monitors the normal chronotrophic response of the heart, i.e. its rate response. But, as is well known, rate is too labile a parameter and can go up and down very quickly and hence can become abnormal on the face of a noxious stimulus and become normal again when that stimulus is off—explaining its false positivity.

Besides, rate is a non-specific response because, ordinarily, fetal heart can primarily respond in only one way irrespective of the nature of the stimulus, i.e. by changing its rate. *So, rate shift in either direction is not specific to hypoxia.*

Endeavors to Look Beyond

Substitute of CTG for Antepartum Fetal Monitoring

Obviously, for monitoring at this period of pregnancy, the technique has to be necessarily external. The two (sort of) alternatives that have been used for the purpose are *biophysical profile scoring* and *Doppler velocimetry*. However, none of these two methods are comparable to CTG as regards the latter's simplicity, ease, versatility, repeatability, portability, price and above all the skill requirement. CTG, in fact, is an essential supplement to these two other techniques and it is finally on the CTG monitoring finding that the final decision to interfere is usually depended upon because it (CTG) gives 'on the spot' (of that minute's) state. To summarise the current position of the various antenatal fetal monitoring techniques available—it may be said that—where the other tests end CTG begins.

Substitute of CTG for Intrapartum Fetal Monitoring

So for over second half of this century, i.e. since 1959 (Hon, 1959) three such methods have come in the clinical scene namely – pH estimation of fetal blood, assay of fetal blood lactate level and fetal oximetry. Of these the first two methods aim to assess whether the fetus has become acidotic or not as a consequence of hypoxia and the third method gives the oxygen saturation of fetal blood.

However, besides many other drawbacks, since the first two methods involve putting incision on the fetal skin and that too repeatedly—these have not become popular.

In any case, these invasive procedures are indicated only when CTG shows pathological tracing which means CTG still remains as the primary method of fetal monitoring.

As regards pulse oximeter, which has the advantage that it does not involve any incision on fetal skin, the oximetry probe has only to be placed just in contact with the intact skin, e.g. over the cheek or the back of the fetus, though has been on trial for over twenty years its reliability has not been established beyond doubt. Besides, though actual incision is not involved, this technique is still fairly intrusive with the *risk of injury* to the fetus, the uterus and even the placenta specially if it is placed posteriorly and more so if it is low. Again, for this method too, it is best to use it as a secondary method to double check pathological CTG traces.

In contrast to all the above three complicated and highly sophisticated techniques of intrapartum monitoring—CTG can do the job completely externally (and also internally by just placement of a scalp electrode). So, from the above review, it is obvious that these methods really are not even a near substitute of CTG.

Beyond CTG—What?

Actually, what we are looking for is a technique with the following features:

- A technique that would measure *both* the oxygen and the acid-base parameters of fetus as desired, specially at the tissue level and particularly that *of the brain tissue.*
- Be non-invasive
- External
- Not painful or uncomfortable for the mother
- Dynamic
- On line
- Clearly objective
- User friendly
- Easily interpretable or Computer interpreted
- Easily repeatable
- 100% dependable
- Safe for both mother and baby
- Should have a reasonable 'lead time', i.e. time for planning action specially arrangement for delivery/ cesarean, etc. if the test shows ominous result

- Should be usable for the purpose of both antepartum and intra-partum fetal monitoring.

  Certainly such an ideal device is not easy to design but endeavor is on as summerised below.

LASER SPECTROSCOPY

It is a revolutionary ingenious German method of measuring fetal oxygen and the related biochemical parameters which uses light energy (as opposed to sound energy like ultrasound). This is however is in experimental stage.

Basis

Spectroscopic observence and analysis of returning laser beams of four different wavelengths in relation to time. It is the changes in optical density and absorbance of light which produces the result.

The Equipment

- Data collection unit—as used for NIRS (Near Infra Red Spectro-scopy) with a dedicated microcomputer board.
- A Laser transmitter board having Laser diodes of 4 pre-set wave-lengths, i.e. 775, 805, 845 and 904.
- A sensor (Probe) having two prisms:
  - A Transmitter prism
  - A Receiver prism
- A receiver module containing:
  - An optical receiver
  - An amplifier
  - A converter
- A standard PC with CPU, Monitor, Printer, etc for the purpose of data processing and graphics

Placement on Patient

All that is required is positioning of the Sensor (Probe) on mother's abdomen over the fetal head, i.e. it is **totally non-invasive**

The Fetal Oxygen Parameters that the Laser Spectroscopy can Display

1. Oxyhemoglobin level
2. Desaturated hemoglobin level
3. Total haemoglobin
4. Cytochrome aa-3 enzyme level

   (Cy aa-3 enzyme or intracellular redox is the final intracellular enzyme that is required for energy metabolism which transfers Hydrogens to Oxygen to form water)

5. Relative change in local 'blood volume'.

The Organ Targeted for this Investigation

It is the fetal brain tissue which is targeted for this investigation because it is the hypoxic damage to the brain that is the primary and acute concern of all.

It is hoped that in near future with further refinement this highly efficient, clearly objective, multiparameter, totally non-invasive technique will be a part of routine fetal monitoring.

FETAL MAGNETOCARDIOGRAPHY (F-MCG)

Scientific Basis of F-MCG

It is a ***noninvasive technique*** of recording *'magnetic fields'* generated by the electrical activity of the fetal heart.

(Unlike fetal MRI, f-MCG ***does not emit*** *magnetic fields* or energy).

It is a 'passive' recording technique, (analogous to the ECG).

It utilises the extremely high sensitivity 'Superconducting Quantum Interference Device' (SQUID) sensors. These sensors amplify signals that are naturally occurring but extremely weak—of the order of 10^{-12} tesla and gives out the detailed electrophysiologic events that is occurring in the fetal heart.

FETAL MONITORING PARAMETERS THAT F-MCG TECHNIQUE CAN PROVIDE TOTALLY NON-INVASIVELY

- Can give fetal ECG parameters unaffected by the presence of vernix in contrast to normal usual f-ECG
- Beat-to-beat fetal heart rate analysis like baseline variability of FHR
  - in normal rhythm as well as
  - in fetal arrhythmias.
- Can be a useful adjunct to electrophysiologic diagnosis of the changes of Fetal heart–like *hidden electrophysiologic disease* such as - QT prolongation, bundle branch block, abnormalities in depolarization and repolarization etc i.e. the mechanisms of fetal cardiac arrhythmias
- Can record fetal movement in detail, i.e. can give good Actocardiography
- Can give fetal heart-CNS interactions – which appear to change in response to stress.

'ABDOMINAL' F-ECG RECORDING THROUGH WIRELESS 'WEARABLE' SYSTEMS

This Italian technique uses—Field Programmable Gate Array (FPGA).

This allows domicillary fetal monitoring and f-ECG is then send to Specialist unit through telephone. The technique is under investigation.

FURTHER READING

1. Beard RW, Filshie GM et al. Significance of the changes in the continuous fetal heart rate in the first stage of labour, J Obstet Gynaecol Brit Cwlth, 1971;78:865–81.

2. Fanelli A, Ferrario M, Piccini L, Andreoni G, Matrone G, Magenes G, Signorini MG.:Prototype of a 'wearable' system for remote fetal monitoring during pregnancy, Politecnico di Milano, Dipartimento di Bioingegneria, Piazza Leonardo da Vinci 32, 20133, Italy. andre. fanelli@mail.polimi.it

3. Hon EH. Obstet Gynec, 1959;14:154.

4. Konje JC and Taylor DJ: Objective Structured Clinical Examination in Obstetrics & Gynaecology,Oxford Blackwell Science, 1998:103.

5. Schmidt S, Gorrissen S et al. Transabdominal Laser Spectroscopy in human fetus during labor, in Perinatology, edited by Saling E, Nestle Nutrition Workshop series, Vevey/Raven Press, New York, 1992, 26:87–93.

6. Schmidt S : Laserspectroscopy in the fetus during labour: Eur J Obstet Gynecol Reprod Biol, 2003 Sep 22;110 Suppl 1:S127–31

7. Strasburger JF, Cheulkar B, and Wakai RT: Magnetocardiography for Fetal Arrhythmias, Author manuscript; available in PMC 2009 July 1, Published in final edited form as: Heart Rhythm. 2008 July; 5(7):1073–6.

CHAPTER 24

Role of CTG for Patients Getting Epidural Analgesia in Labor

Here is a startling statistics—About 10% patients receiving epidural analgesia show FHR abnormality on CTG specially decelerations.

MECHANISM OF CAUSATION OF FHR ABNORMALITY
By Causing Maternal Hypotension
This is brought about by the effect of epidural on maternal autonomic nervous system (sympathetic block) and this hypotension is most marked in utero-placental circulation. The latter point is evidenced by the finding that blood pressure in femoral artery is often found to be 20 mm lower than that in the brachial artery after epidural block.

This can lead to hypoxia, and FHR abnormality occurs as an effect of hypoxia. Sometimes however, 20 to 30 minutes after top up , there is fetal bradycardia without any obvious maternal hypotension. This may be due to re-distribution of maternal blood volume (Steer, 1986).

By Quinidine Like Effect of Local Anesthetic Agents (Caine Drugs) on Fetal Myocardium
The local anesthetic agents get rapidly absorbed from extradural space into maternal circulation—and affects fetal myocardium (Beard, 1974).

In this regard, Flynn and Kelly (1982) explained that fetus may not suffer from any morbidity during the period of deceleration induced by caine drugs as long as fetus remains within the uterus until the deceleration is resolved. Morbidity will result if the fetus is delivered prior to the time when the caine drug has been metabolised by the fetus (usually between 8–16 minutes).

By Causing Pyrexia

It has been found that epidural causes rise of temperature by an average of 1°C per 10 hours by causing reduced heat loss through paralysis of autonomic nerves preventing sweating (Steer, 1986). This pyrexia may be associated with fetal tachycardia.

Aorta-Caval Compression

Patients getting epidural analgesia, if kept in supine position for any length of time, the consequent aortocaval compression contributes further to the hypotension of epidural per se.

Increased Uterine Activity

This may be occasioned by epidural and also can sometimes contribute to FHR abnormality.

However, it must be emphasized here that with skilled anesthetist and close supervision the complications mentioned above are rather rare.

TYPES OF FHR ABNORMALITY

Short episodes of tachycardia, deep deceleration, prolonged deceleration, late deceleration and loss of beat-to-beat variation etc. (Beard, 1974, William's Obstetrics, 2010) have all been reported with epidural analgesia.

Likely Clinical Causes for FHR Abnormality

- Excessive dose
- Too rapid pushing of the drug
- Administration of epidural with patient in wrong position.

Management of Abnormal CTG Trace due to Caine Drugs

- Fluid loading (Hartman's solution)—specially preloading as a prevention.
- Repositioning of the mother.
- Oxygen inhalation.

These measures are usually sufficient to restore the fetal heart rate to normal.

Recommendation

In view of the above, epidural analgesia in labor should always be given under cover of CTG (Desouza and Arulkumaran, 2009).

FURTHER READING

1. Beard RW. Fetal heart rate patterns and their clinical interpretation. Sonicaid Ltd., Bognor Regis, Sussex, UK, 1974;1–56.
2. D'Souza R and Arulkumaran S: 'Intrapartum Fetal Surveillance' in the book Best Practice in Labor and Delivery, Edited by Warren R and Arulkumaran S, 2009;38–53.
3. Flynn AM, Kelly J. Recent Advances in Obst. and Gynaec, Edited by Bonnar J, Churchill Livingstone 1982;14:25–45.
4. Steer PJ. Fetal heart rate patterns and their clinical interpretation. Oxford Sonicaid Ltd, Sussex, UK, 1986;1–44.
5. William's Obstetrics: 23rd edition, Edited by Cunningham FG, Leveno KJ, Bloom SL, Hauth JC, Rouse DJ and Spong CY, Intrapartum Assessment, Mc Graw Hill, New York, 2010;424, 456.

Effects of Narcotic Drugs on CTG

A large variety of Central Nervous System (CNS) depressant drugs have been found to cause transient diminished beat-to-beat variability, for example –Narcotics, Barbiturates, Phenothiazines, Tranquilizers, Meperidine, Butorphenol etc (William's Obstetrics, 2010).
Here is some details on some commonly used drugs.

Magnesium Sulphate

Diminished baseline variability and also blunted frequency of accelerations have been reported with the infusion of Magnesium Sulphate after three hour of use (William's Obstetrics, 2010).

Diazepam

Please *see* **Figure 13.41**. It clearly demonstrates the effects of Diazepam 10 mg. IV on a hypertensive antenatal patient at 36 weeks. Within two minutes of the injection—the beat-to-beat variability flatened. It has been observed by the author that it sometimes takes 30 minutes or more for the beat-to-beat variation to normalize.

If this flat CTC causes worry, a quick Vibroacoustic stimulation test (VAST) may be done and, if the fetus is not basically compromised—it will respond to the stimulation in spite of Diazepam effect—though may be just momentarily. One spurt of VAST does not often cure the diminished variability in such cases. Anyway, it is best to do at least 10 minutes NST before giving the Diazepam injection to check the prevailing baseline FHR of the fetus to avoid undue worry later. However, it is really not necessary to give VAST in such cases because the cause is known.

Pethidine

Pethidine given even in therapeutic doses (100 mg) can cause the following FHR abnormalities—reduced baseline variability often making it almost a straight line, slight decrease in baseline FHR (by 10–12 BPM) and reduced number and amplitude of FH accelerations (*see* **Fig. 13.40**). Besides, it also reduces the fetal activity as can be easily seen in actogram. Hence, ideally, to avoid confusion, it is better to do a 10 minutes tracing before giving injection of any narcotic drug. The effect of the drug is expected to get reversed by 1 hour. However, if the tracing is causing worry—its antidote Naloxone may be given and the tracing observed to see, whether the undesirable CTG changes are getting reversed or not. Further course of action is decided according to the finding of this therapeutic test.

FURTHER READING

1. Beard RW. Fetal Heart Rate Patterns and their Clinical Interpretation. Published by Sonicaid Limited Bognor Regis, Sussex, UK, 1974;44–45.
2. Ingemarsson I, Ingemarsson E, Spencer JAD. Fetal Heart Rate Monitoring: A Practical Guide, Oxford University Press, Oxford, 1993;265–69.
3. William's Obstetrics: 23rd edition, Edited by Cunningham FG, Leveno KJ, Bloom SL, Hauth JC, Rouse DJ and Spong CY, Intrapartum Assessment, Mc Graw Hill, New York, 2010;417.

CHAPTER 26

Special Problems of CTG Monitoring of Preterm Pregnancy

This implies the problem of interpretation of FHR pattern of fetuses of gestational age under 36 weeks and certainly of those under 34 weeks.

NORMAL PATTERN

The criteria for normal pattern before 32 to 34 weeks is not yet clearly established. However, this is what can be roughly concluded from available data:

Baseline Rate and Baseline Variability

Baseline tachycardia and reduced baseline variability is a common finding in preterm pregnancy. This is due to immaturity of the vagal centre which, as has been proved, matures progressively as the gestation progresses. This constitutes a major source of confusion in diagnosis of hypoxia in these fetuses.

Sleep-Activity Cycle

This cycle of perterm fetuses is of short duration of 10 minutes each in contrast to that of fetuses near term in which this cycle is usually of 30 minutes duration and particularly the sleep period in these cases very rarely exceeds 40 minutes (Ingemarsson et al, 1993).

Fetal Movement

Though the number of fetal movement is more during preterm period, these are less strong and lasts for a very short duration. This, to some extent, explains the poor reactivity of preterm fetus (see below).

Response of FHR to Fetal Movement

Between 25–30 weeks decelerations (rather than acceleration) are more common with FM and they are usually of the amplitude of 15–30 BPM and lasts for 15 to 30 seconds. Decelerations disappear and FM acceleration (reactivity) starts as the fetus approaches term (Ingemarsson et al, 1993).

Variable Deceleration

This occurs in 70% of preterm fetuses between 28 to 30 weeks and in 50% of those that are even of higher maturity than above (Ingemarsson et al, 1993).

ABNORMAL PATTERN

Tachycardia and Reduced Variability

As already mentioned, these criteria when present, are difficult to interpret because these are often not associated with fetal acidosis in preterm fetus.

'Absent' Variability, Late Deceleration and Combined Deceleration (i.e. Variable Plus Late Deceleration)

These patterns are more commonly associated with acidosis even in preterm fetuses. The clinical background of these cases i.e., whether the fetus is growth retarded, whether there is associated oligohydramnios, whether the patient is hypertensive, is diabetic, whether it is a case of premium pregnancy etc. should be given critical consideration for taking decision.

REVISED DEFINITION OF ACCELERATION FOR PRE-TERM PREGNANCY

For gestation before 32 weeks of pregnancy – it is rise in FHR by 10 beats per minute lasting for at least 10 seconds (National Institute of Child Health and Human development—Fetal Monitoring Workshop, 1997).

SPECIAL RISKS OF FHR ABNORMALITIES FOR PRETERM FETUSES

In preterm fetuses (specially under 34 weeks) hypoxia and acidosis can aggravate respiratory distress syndrome (RDS) and may contribute to intraventricular hemorrhage and its sequelae warrenting early action in presence of an abnormal trace (D'Souza R and Arulkumaran, 2009).

FURTHER READING

1. D'Souza R and Arulkumaran S: 'Intrapartum Fetal Surveillance' in the book Best Practice in Labor and Delivery, Edited by Warren R and Arulkumaran S, 2009;49.
2. Ingemarsson I, Ingemarsson E, Spencer JAD. Fetal Heart Rate Monitoring—A Practical Guide. Oxford University press, 1993;213–22.
3. National Institute of Child Health and Human development—Fetal Monitoring Workshop, 1997: Electronic Fetal Heart Monitoring: Research Guideline for Interpretation, Am J Obstet Gynecol, 1997;177:1385.
4. William's Obstetrics: 23rd edition, Edited by Cunningham FG, Leveno KJ, Bloom SL, Hauth JC, Rouse DJ and Spong CY, Intrapartum Assessment, Mc Graw Hill, New York, 2010;338.

Monitoring Twins by CTG

- Non-Invasive Monitoring
- Invasive Monitoring

NON-INVASIVE MONITORING

This is done abdominally with the help of two US transducers of two different frequencies, one of 1.5 MHZ and one of 2 MHZ. One of these is placed over the heart of one fetus and the other over the heart of the other fetus. Of course, for this kind of dual monitoring, CTG machine with 'dual FH' monitoring capability is required, i.e. the machine should have two sockets for the two (Ultrasonic) FH transducers.

One can have FHR tracing of two fetuses either one above the other (in which case a special tracing paper in which the FHR channel has been divided into halves—upper and lower with condensed calibration is required (**Fig. 27.1**) or have tracing of both fetuses together on the standard CTG paper (commonly used). In the latter case usually the two traces are of two tones—one darker than the other and so are quite easy to identify.

Caution

One must make sure that one is recording two different heart rates!

Non-invasive monitoring can be used for both antepartum and intrapartum monitoring.

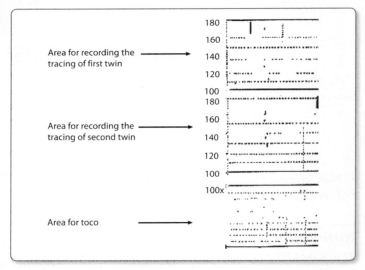

Fig. 27.1 This is a photocopy of a 'special' CTG tracing paper meant for recording FHR tracing of two fetuses of twins seperately. In this the normal FHR area of the CTG paper has been divided into two halves—upper and lower and FHR range between 100 to 180 BPM has been printed twice in this area once in the upper-half and once in the lower-half by condensing the gaps between the BPM increment lines. These are no longer used

INVASIVE MONITORING

This is meant only for the first twin in labor with ruptured membranes. The presenting fetus can be monitored by placement of electrode on its body, i.e. internal mode of CTG. Here, obviously, second twin has to be monitored by external mode with abdominal US transducer (**Fig. 27.2**). For this kind of monitoring, i.e. first twin by internal mode, and second twin by external mode, one would need machine with this kind of dual monitoring capability, i.e. facility for both F-ECG and US mode of computation of FHR.

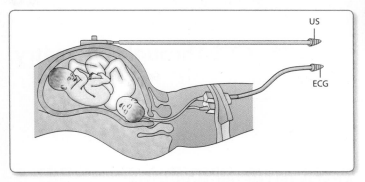

Fig. 27.2 Twins monitoring in labor—first twin being monitored through scalp electrode and second twin by ultrasonic abdominal transducer

PROBLEM OF MONITORING TWINS BY CTG IN LABOR

The CTG procedure here is associted with very high rate of signal loss –

- in First stage – 33%
- in Second stage – 60% (Walkinshaw S, 2009)

FURTHER READING

1. Sonicaid TEAM Fetal Monitor—User's Guide. Publication No. 8909–8500, Issue– 2, 1 Kimber Road, Oxford, UK, 1996;45–60.
2. Walkinshaw S : Breech and Twin delivery, in Best Practice in Labor and Delivery, Edited by Warren R and Arulkumaran S, 2009;125, 126.
3. William's Obstetrics: 23rd edition, Edited by Cunningham FG, Leveno KJ, Bloom SL, Hauth JC, Rouse DJ and Spong CY, Intrapartum Assessment, Mc Graw Hill, New York, 2010;410–43.

CHAPTER **28**

CTG Through Telemetry

WHAT IS TELEMETRIC MONITORING?

Telemetric monitoring means monitoring from a distance. In the present context, in gross practical terms, it means electronic fetal monitoring without any visible physical cable connection between the patient and the CTG machine.

Types of Telemetric Monitoring

Two Types

Telemetry through radio-transmitter This works only within the transmission zone of a transmitter, e.g. within the hospital premises. Its main application is for patients in labor but they being located not in one place (e.g. in labor room), but at many different places within the hospital e.g. in the ward, in the common room, in the hospital garden and, of course, some also in labor room.

Telemetry through telephone line In this mode patient situated at very distant places, e.g. at their home can be monitored from a base station, e.g. specialist obstetric unit through telephone line. Its main application is for antepartum fetal monitoring of high-risk cases.

Procedure of Transmitter Telemetry

This type of telemetry uses the principle of radio-transmission. The system consists of three components and it works like this:

Transmitter

This is a small (walkman size), lightweight, battery operated equipment with a carrying strap which the patient carries around slung from her shoulder like a sash. It has the following sockets:

a. Socket for taking the wires coming from scalp electrode—for fetal ECG.

b. Socket for the cable coming from the intrauterine pressure transducer—for monitoring uterine activity and

c. Socket for mother's remote event marker which is meant for recording her own perception of fetal movement and may be uterine contraction. For recording FHR and contraction by external method the corresponding socket may be used.

Each transmitter (sender) unit is tuned to a 'matched' frequency receiver to avoid interference with other radio units.

Receiver

It's function is to receive the transmitted wave through its antenna. It is usually sited on the top of the CTG machine.

CTG Machine

The receiver, in turn, is connected to the CTG machine for the actual monitoring and giving out the findings and tracings.

Procedure of Telephonic CTG Telemetry

For this, a modem is required just like that for e-mail.

Obstetric nurse visits patients at their homes with a portable CTG machine. She fixes the US and toco transducer on patients' abdomen as usual and starts the machine. The output of the machine is connected to the normal telephone line of patients' home via the modem.

It is so arranged that on switching on, the machine records the events for a pre-set period at the end of which, in auto mode, a specific telephone number (that of the base unit) gets automatically dialed and the data gets automatically transferred to the base machine at the hospital through this telephone. In manual mode, the same thing happens on pressing the 'SEND' switch. In every case, for identification, patients' registration number has to be keyed in first.

As all CTG tracings must be assessed on the background of patients clinical history, the 'analysed' CTG data should ideally be fed in a computer which already has patients' full clinical history stored in it. Sonicaid TEAM fetal monitor, when connected to the Sonicaid AXIS central review system, can receive and display obstetric record from upto 36 fetal monitors at a single point.

Advantages of Telemetry

During Labor

1. Patient can move about at will and need not be tied to a bed.
2. Patient feels more relaxed—not being surrounded by machines.
3. Allows monitoring in transit, e.g. while transferring the patient from labor room to operation room, e.g. for emergency cesarean section.
4. Allows more bedside access; as the machine and it's connecting cables are not around—the attending staff can move freely around the patient.
5. Reduces load on labour ward. If labor ward gets overloaded, some patients can be kept in the low dependency area like ward while still being monitored by labor room staff through telemetry.
6. From a central location, one senior staff can view and monitor the state of fetus of a number of ambulatory patients.
7. It may even help in progress of labor because with this technique the patient is allowed to sit erect, stand and even walk about. An erect posture has been shown to reduce the duration of labor.

During Antenatal Period

Patients who need frequent monitoring like IUGR cases, cases of post dated pregnancy, that of previous stillbirth, etc. can have their monitoring done right at their own home and have the benefit of their data analysed by the specialist at hospital. This saves them the botheration of coming repeatedly to hospital for monitoring and, for some, of the inconvenience and expenditure of getting admitted to hospital for monitoring.

This is also an extremely desirable method of monitoring uterine irritability in the cases who had one or more premature birth in the past.

SOME NEWER MODELS

Basic Technology

Aquires electro-physiological signals of fetal heart *that can be 'passively' detected* by electrodes positioned '*on the maternal abdomen*' thereby monitors 'Fetal ECG' completely externally – under investigation.

Features

- Wearable
- Wireless—requires no wires to connect—to a display or printer.

Advantages

- No need for the constant re-positioning of transducers
- Works well in obese women
- Gives high levels of patient satisfaction.
- Very simple to use
- Globally accessible services at patient's home and hospital

(British model—Beacon by Monica; Italian prototype)

FURTHER READING

1. "Beacon by Monica" sims@launchsomething.com, Monitoring of fetal ECG externally through mothers abdomen.

2. Fanelli A, Ferrario M, Piccini L et al.:Prototype of a 'wearable' system for remote fetal monitoring during pregnancy in domocilliary context, Politecnico di Milano, Dipartimento di Bioingegneria, Piazza Leonardo da Vinci 32, 20133, Italy. andre.fanelli@mail.polimi.it.

3. Hewlett Packard Publication—"Telemetry for Obstetrics" November, Printed in the Federal Republic of Germany, Boblingen 1978.

4. Sonicaid TEAM fetal monitor—User's guide: Publication No. 8909-8500, Issue–2, 1 Kimber Road, Oxford, UK, 1996;99–111.

Clinical Considerations in Interpretation of Abnormal Trace and its Management

CTG is merely an investigative procedure and like all investigations it has its limitations. In any case one cannot treat just an investigation report—one has to treat the whole patient and hence is the necessity to know the full clinical picture of the patient under investigation and use the report in that context.

Factors that need special consideration in case of an abnormal tracing:

- Clinical indication of doing CTG
- Maturity of the fetus
- State of maternal pulse
- State of maternal temperature
- Posture of the patient in which CTG was taken
- Any congenital fetal malformation
- Volume of liquor
- Inducability (in an antenatal case)
- Colour of liquor
- Whether the patient is on oxytocic
- Whether the patient is on continuous epidural analgesia
- Whether she has recently received any centrally acting tranquilizer, sedative or analgesic
- Position of fetal head – Occiputo-anterior/posterior
- Stage of labor and expected time of delivery
- Presence of any of the following complications of labor like dehydration, ketosis, etc.
- Results of other fetal monitoring tests.

Clinical Indication of Doing CTG

This is the first thing that one has to ascertain before giving the final judgement on an abnormal tracing. It is one thing if it is coming from a low-risk or no-risk patient, i.e. one having absolutely no clinical abnormality (like a CTG done as a routine screening procedure on a young healthy normotensive primigravida at 38th week of pregnancy) and it is quite a different thing getting the same abnormal patch from a high-risk case like one of IUGR, post-dated pregnancy, APH, pregnancy induced hypertension, etc.

Not only this, the gravity and tempo of the risk factor also should be given due consideration, e.g. severity of growth retardation, level of blood pressure and degree of proteinuria, number of bleed and amount of bleeding in a case of APH, degree of postmaturity (days past), etc. (*see* the 'Risk Classification' in Chapter 17).

Maturity of the Fetus

About the *postdated pregnancy*—mention has already been made above. The specific point to remember here is—FHR between 100–120 BPM may be considered as normal in a post-term fetus provided the baseline variability remains normal, FHR shows qualifying acceleration with fetal movement and there is no deceleration (Steer, 1986).

As regards *pre-term pregnancy*—CTG tracings at this maturity are very difficult to interpret and needs exercising of great caution. This is because baseline tachycardia and reduced baseline variability is a common finding in normal pre-term pregnancy and FHR does not always accelerate with FM—may even decelerate (see Chapter 26—Special Problems of CTG Monitoring of Preterm Pregnancy).

State of Maternal Pulse

As regards baseline tachycardia, it should be remembered that the chemicals in maternal blood which induces maternal tachycardia can also, logically, cause fetal tachycardia. So, in all cases of fetal baseline tachycardia, maternal pulse must be counted for full 1 minute.

In the case of fetal baseline bradycardia also maternal pulse must be checked as a matter of routine because US transducer can easily pick up pulse of maternal aorta instead of FHS which may pass as fetal bradycardia and patient may end up in an unnecessary cesarean section for false fetal distress. Through the same mechanism a case of intrauterine death may be falsely diagnosed as one of live fetus having baseline bradycardia (*see* **Figs 13.47 and 13.48**).

To differentiate fetal heart signal from maternal heart signal all that one has to do is—put a finger on maternal pulse and judge whether its rhythm is synchronous with that of the audible FHS sound from the CTG machine or not. Normally, FHS and maternal pulse should be asynchronous. Alternatively, putting the FH transducer over mother's heart for 1 minute solves the problem immediately.

Maternal tachycardia associated with severe maternal anemia and heart failure may also be associated with fetal baseline tachycardia.

State of Maternal Temperature

Maternal pyrexia due to whatever cause can induce both maternal and fetal tachycardia as already mentioned.

Posture of the Patient in which CTG was Taken

The posture in which the tracing has been taken is also of some importance because *supine hypotension* can give abnormal tracing which is correctable by simply turning the patient on her side.

Besides, some *cord compression* can get released by change of maternal posture and this must be tried in all cases specially in those of variable deceleration.

Any Congenital Fetal Malformation

In all cases of abnormal tracing, fetal CNS malformation must always be kept in mind. If it has not been excluded already by previous ultrasound scan, a quick intranatal scan should be done to exclude this before taking the patient up for cesarean section.

Colour Doppler plus Echcardiography of fetal heart can exclude fetal congenital heart block *in suspected cases*.

Volume of Liquor

In the cases with clinically suspected oligohydramnios, more so if it has been further confirmed by measurement of amniotic fluid index (less than 5), CTG abnormality should be taken very seriously.

Oligohydramnios, besides in itself being a sign of placental insufficiency, increases the chance of cord compression between the fetal body and the uterine wall or in-between the folds of fetal limbs, as described under 'variable deceleration' in Chapter 12 amnioinfusion can reverse CTG abnormalities due to cord compression associated with oligohydramnios.

Inducability

In high-risk cases with suspicious CTG, if Bishop's score is good, if 3/5 or less portion of head is palpable per abdomen (i.e. if the presenting part is not high) and if fetus is mature enough, in author's view, one should plan to deliver such a case rather than waiting (or rather pushing the fetus) until the tracing becomes abnormal and then do the induction (and end up doing emergency CS for fetal distress.

Color of Liquor

Abnormal FHR pattern has been reported to be more common with thick meconium stained amniotic fluid (Arulkumaran, 1992). Further, it has also been found that the incidence of low Apgar trebles with this omnious combination of thick meconium and abnormal tracing (Steer, 1989).

Whether the Patient is on Oxytocic

This applies to the patient whose labor is being induced or augmented by oxytocin drip or prostaglandin. The cause of abnormal trace in these cases may be uterine hypertonus, its polysystole, occurrence of prolonged contraction, etc. Reduction of drip rate or complete stoppage of oxytocic often normalises the tracing in these cases.

Whether the Patient is on Continuous Epidural Analgesia

About 10% of patients receiving epidural analgesia have been reported to show FHR abnormality on CTG (see chapter 24—"Role of CTG for Patient's getting Epidural Analgesia in Labor").

Whether She has Recently Received any Centrally Acting Tranquilizer, Sedative or Analgesic

It is well known that these may cause reduced baseline variability, diminished fetal movement and reduced frequency of acceleration (William's Obstetrics, 2010).

Position of Fetal Head

For patients in labor this is of relevance because incidence of variable deceleration has been found to be nearly double (59.4% in comparison to 32.8% in OA position) with occipito-posterior (OP) position although the frequency of fetal acidaemia was not found to be any higher in this group in comparison to OA position group. This FH pattern in OP position is thought to be due to compression of fetal head in its deflexed posture as is often the case with OP position (Ingemarsson et al, 1993).

Stage of Labor and Expected Time of Delivery

This is a vital point because on it depends whether to deliver the patient immediately or to give her some time under close observation so that the patient progresses further and normal vaginal delivery is possible.

Presence of any of the Following Complications of Labor Like Dehydration, Ketosis, etc.

These conditions are often associated with both maternal and fetal tachycardia. So, these, when present, should be promptly corrected while monitoring should be continued to see whether tachycardia gets corrected by this means or not.

Results of Other Fetal Monitoring Tests

For an antenatal case, the tracing character should be correlated with AFI score, Doppler velocimetry finding and biophysical profile if the patient had any of these done.

For a patient in labor, abnormal tracing should be correlated with fetal ECG recording, pulse oxymetry (Seelbach-Gobel and Dildy, 1999) and scalp pH / Lactate value if these have been done.

FURTHER READING

1. Arulkumaran S. Obstetrics and Gynaecology for postgraduates, 1st edn, Edited by Ratnam SS, Bhaskar Rao K, Arulkumaran S. Orient Longman, Madras, India, 1992;115–26.
2. D'Souza R, Arulkumaran S. 'Intrapartum Fetal Surveillance' in the book Best Practice in Labor and Delivery, Edited by Warren R and Arulkumaran S, 2009;38–53.
3. Edwin C, Arulkumaran S. Electronic fetal heart monitoring in current & future practice, The Journal of O & G of India, Vol 58, 2008;121–30.
4. Ingemarsson I, Ingemarsson E, Spencer JAD. Fetal Heart Monitoring—A Practical Guide. Oxford University Press, Oxford, 1993;178–79.
5. Magowan B, Owen P, Drife J: Clinical Obst Gynae, 2nd edition, Monitoring the fetus in labor, Elsevier, Edinburgh, 2009;331–43.
6. NICE (National Institute for Clinical Excellance) Guideline :The Clinical Guideline No. 70, Induction of labour, RCOG press, 2008, London
7. Seelbach-Gobel B, Dildy GA. Fetal pulse oxymetry and other monitoring modalities. Clinics in Perinatology 1999;26(4):881–91.
8. Steer PJ. Fetal heart rate patterns and their clinical interpretations. Oxford Sonicaid Ltd, Sussex, UK, 1986;1–44.
9. Steer PJ. Obstet Gynecol 1986;74:715–21.
10. William's Obstetrics: 23rd edition, Edited by Cunningham FG, Leveno KJ, Bloom SL, Hauth JC, Rouse DJ and Spong CY, Intrapartum Assessment, Mc Graw Hill, New York, 2010;410–43

CHAPTER 30

Medicolegal Consideration of CTG

Symonds (1994) reported that 70% of all liability claims related to brain damage are based on reputed abnormality of fetal heart rate tracing on CTG.

While on one hand CTG tracing may save obstetricians from trouble in some cases of false blame put on them for wrong fetal management, on the other hand it necessitates the Obstetrician to be even more careful about his action and inaction because the tracing constitutes a hard objective evidence of the events.

How Long CTG Tracings must be Kept Saved?

For medicolegal purpose, CTG tracing must be kept for 25 years (Fraser and Cooper, 2009).

How to Store CTG Tracings?

Electronic System/Paperless System

The advantages of this system of storing are –
- Huge amount of data can be kept in almost *no physical space*
- *Easy instant retrieval* in few seconds
- Excellent for *Audit and research*
- 'on-line' saving, i.e. as and when CTG being done is possible. This is the ideal system.

Physical Storage

It is full of disadvantages as detailed below;

- Needs huge space
- Retrieval very difficult
- Tracings done on thermal papers fades within a few months. This is not recommended.

    Tracings should be at least stored in CD or Pendrive.

There is also another system of storage called WORM (Write Once Read Many-times). This uses optical disks and can archive upto 4000 cases of average tracing duration of 8 hours (D'Souza and Arulkumaran, 2009).

CTG with On-line 'Computer Analysis' Facility

These machines are a boon for medicolegal purpose because here the 'interpretation and the diagnosis' given by the machine is also automatically saved (Laybourn and Mander, 2000; Edwin and Arulkumaran, 2008) unlike the conventional visual analysis system where these are to be first done manually and then anoted on the tracing. Currently such computer analysis facility is available for antepartum CTG tracings only.

Double Checking an Abnormal Trace

Wherever possible, abnormal tracing is best double-checked by VAST which is applicable for both antenatal and also intranatal cases. For antenatal traces in particular—biophysical profile, Doppler velocimetry are the two options and for labor cases—F-ECG, Fetal blood sampling and pH or Lactate estimation. Results of these are also to be written on the CTG trace paper.

Some Precautionary Steps to Avoid Litigation on Fetal Monitoring by CTG

- Time (from and to) the CTG was done must be written on the acutal tracing. Newer machine automatically prints it. This is vital because judgement on timing of intervention, of delays, etc. is judged on these.

- Some models have serial number printed on the paper at every 10 minutes and this also checked if there is a law suit.
- In the cases of intermittent CTG monitoring, which is often the case, clinical auscultation with fetoscope or Doptone whenever it is done in the in-between time must also be recorded with time.
- If several stripes of CTG have been taken at various times—these should be numbered chronologically and serially as 1, 2, 3, 4, etc. so that evolution can be assessed.
- No bit of tracing must be thrown away without analysing.
- If possible get all tracings analysed by an expert/senior. The modern telemetry facility through telephone link can make the latter easily possible. But the expert must write his or her final interptretation/ opinion *on the tracing* like – NORMAL/NON-REASSURING/ ABNORMAL and sign with date and time.
- Important management events must also be written on the tracing paper like – time of PV, of Epidural or its top-up, of FBS, etc.
- Patient's name and her Hostipal registration No. has to be written on the tracing otherwise it is not a valid evidence.

AUTHOR'S VIEW

The author believes that court room is not the right or the proper place to make scientific judgement on a FHR tracing. An undelivered patient in hand is a very different atmosphere, circumstance and mental stress than the situation once the delivery has taken place by whatever means – a diffused situation. Yet, unfortunately, many retrospective judgements are passed against FHR measurements by CTG in legal suits.

FURTHER READING

1. Carter MC, Steer PJ. Brit J Obstet Gynaecol 1993;100(Supple)9:2.
2. D'Souza R, Arulkumaran S. 'Intrapartum fetal surveillance' in the book Best Practice in Labor and Delivery, Edited by Warren R and Arulkumaran S, 2009;38–53.

3. Edwin C, Arulkumaran S. Electronic fetal heart monitoring in current & future practice, The Journal of O & G of India, Vol 58, 2008;121–130.

4. Fraser DM, Cooper MA. In Myles' Textbook for Midwives, 15th ed, 2009; 481-4.

5. Laybourn M, Mander AM. Progress in obstetrics and gynaecology. Studd J 2000;14:188–201.

6. Symonds EM. Fetal monitoring—Medical and legal implications for the practitioners. Current opinion. Obstet Gynecol 1994;6:430.

Drawbacks and Deficiencies of CTG Monitoring

Though CTG has found wide acceptance throughout the world it has certain drawbacks and deficiencies which can be discussed under the following headings:

- Difficulty in interpretation
- High false positive rate
- Causes other than hypoxia producing abnormal tracing
- CTG brings about increase in interference rate
- Reduces human contact and interaction with patient
- The procedure induces unnecessary fear complex in the mind of the mother.

Difficulty in Interpretation

This has been discussed in detail in Chapter 14—"Problems in interpretation of CTG and solutions", Chapter 22—"Non-reassuring CTG trace" and Chapter 23—"Beyond CTG".

But difficulty in interpretation is perhaps not all that great as shown by the result of the following study; "trained observers will agree on abnormal and normal fetal heart traces, however defined, on 87 occasions out of 100. This is a good agreement, suggesting that electronic fetal monitoring is a reliable test (Grant, 1999).

However, significant interpretation problem remains in the following two areas:

- Tracing from a pre-term fetus—Tracings from fetuses of under 36, more so under 34 weeks of gestation is still difficult to interpret in spite of the auto analysis facility the reasons of which have been described in Chapter 26—"Special Problems of CTG Monitoring of Preterm Pregnancy".

- Tracing of second stage of labor—Peculiarly, high incidence of variable deceleration (33%) or an unclassifiable pattern (36%) have been reported in literature at this stage of labor (Stone and Murray, 1995) which poses difficult interpretation problems. But, usually these cases are not very difficult to manage since in most of these the delivery is imminent. However, if in any patient the second stage is found to be getting prolonged and the case is also showing such FHR abnormality a F-ECG cum STAN or FBS and pH or Lactate estimation is indicated if such facilities are available otherwise arrangement should be made to expedite the delivery (also see under Chapter 33—the heading "Special features of CTG monitoring in second stage").

High False Positive Rate

As already mentioned conventional CTG, both antenatal and intranatal, have been reported to have roughly 50% false positivity rate, i.e. abnormal tracing but unaffected fetus. This constitutes the major cause of high interference rate with the use of CTG monitoring. The solution to this has been described in details in Chapter 23—"Beyond CTG".

Causes Other than Hypoxia Producing Abnormal Tracing

These have been described in detail under Chapter 15 in the section "Non-stress Test". These cause, almost all of these being of simple clinical nature like—maternal tachycardia, maternal pyrexia, maternal sedation, use of epidural, presence of dehydration and ketosis, maternal position (supine or lateral), maturity of the fetus, etc. are by no means difficult to spot. All that is required is the awareness and knowledge about the inter-relation between these clinical parameters and CTG tracing. This has been described point by point in Chapter 29—"Clinical Considerations in Interpretation of Abnormal Trace and its Management".

CTG brings about Increase in Interference Rate

Leveno et al (1986) reported that electronic fetal monitoring increases the diagnosis of fetal distress in both high- and low-risk pregnancies and thereby increases the rate of cesarean section without perinatal benefit as measured by customary neonatal morbidity criteria. In 690 high-risk patients under randomised controlled trial their cesarean section rate was 6% for auscultation, 18% for electronic fetal monitoring by CTG and 11% for CTG plus FBS and pH estimation. From the above result it would appear that in 7% cases CTG overdiagnosed fetal distress but more importantly *in 5% cases auscultation missed fetal distress*—as proved by fetal FBS and pH estimation.

The conclusion the above result would lend is—CTG certainly has a definite place in fetal monitoring in labor, however, it also does increase the interference rate unless abnormal tracing cases are double checked by methods like F-ECG, FBS and VAST.

CTG Reduces Human Contact and Interaction with Patient

This, need not at all be so, provided human beings present in labor room has inclination and time for it.

CTG Induces Unnecessary Fear Complex in the Mind of the Mother

Some group have suggested that gadgetory monitoring of labor with belts, wires, pipes issuing from the patient and going to machine tends to depict the process of labor as an abnormal affair rather than a physiological process thereby breeds unnecessary fear complex in the minds of mother.

Contrary to this, the author in his survey of 500 patients about their attitude about CTG monitoring during labor found *over 90% considered it greatly reassuring and welcomed—even requested for it.*

FURTHER READING

1. Grant JM. 'The reliability of electronic fetal monitoring'. Brit J Obst Gynaec Editorial, 1999;7–8.
2. Leveno KJ, Cunningham FG, Nelson S, Roark Micki, et al. N Engl J Med 1986;315:615–9.
3. Stone PR, Murray HG. John Bonnar (Ed). Recent Advances in Obst Gynec. London: Churchill Livingstone. 1995;19:45–62.
4. Strachan B. 'The Management of intrapartum Fetal Distress' in the book Best Practice in Labor and Delivery, Edited by Warren R, Arulkumaran S, 2009;66–75.
5. William's Obstetrics: 23rd edition, Edited by Cunningham FG, Leveno KJ, Bloom SL, Hauth JC, Rouse DJ and Spong CY, Intrapartum Assessment, Mc Graw Hill, New York, 2010;410–43.

32

Place of CTG Today

UNIVERSAL MONITORING

It is now established that 'routine' monitoring of 'all' pregnancies and 'all' labors (continuously) including the enormous number of 'low risk cases' by CTG is not useful, would be extremely expensive and may actually be counterproductive because such practice is known to increase operative delivery rate greatly without corresponding improvement in fetal, neonatal or post-neonatal result. So, it boils down that, to be beneficial, only around 30 percent of pregnant population, i.e. those who have some risk factors should be monitored by CTG.

SELECTIVE MONITORING

However, a disquieting point still remains about the above policy of selective monitoring specially in the case of intrapartum monitoring in that—fetal distress, fetal death and postnatal morbidities also do occur, though with less frequency, even in the low risk cases. So, the question arises how to prevent these untowards events in these unsuspecting cases.

Then there is the problem—*How to justify*, when challenged by a patient who has suffered such a loss, for not using the monitor on her particularly when this facility was available in the unit. In these situations, practice of this even very logical conservatism becomes a major issue and comes under attack (such problems have been faced by the author).

As already described, use of '*Admission test*' specially with the application of Vibroacoustic stimulation (VAST) could be a way out for screening low risk intrapartum cases specially when they are unbooked or had inadequate antenatal care and where work load of the hospital is high. This way the expense of monitoring will be minimum considering the cover it will give to a large number.

In the following section the position of CTG has been examined in great detail to seek out its real place both for antepartum and also for intrapartum monitoring.

ANTENATAL CTG—CRITICAL APPRAISAL

FIGO news (1987) recommends that antepartum electronic FH monitoring should be used for diagnostic (screening) purposes only and the results should be interpreted in context of the clinical indication of performing the test, i.e. in the context of prevailing risk factors and their severity in any individual case. This is justifiable in view of the fact that positive predictive value of a non-reactive antepartum CTG had been reported as only 50 percent (Low et al, 1986).

However, as we know today that this false positivity rate can be greatly reduced by the *application of Vibroacoustic stimulation* (VAST) with CTG.

In selected antenatal cases, specially where placental insufficiency is strongly suspected, e.g. in the cases of gross IUGR, of post-dated pregnancy of over 1 week's duration and, of course, in all the cases where oligohydramnios is suspected—amniotic fluid index (AFI) estimation is a desired adjunct and so is **Doppler** velocimetry and S/D ratio assessment.

Actually the real value of antepartum CTG monitoring lies in its extremely low false negative rate, i.e. if all parameters of CTG is excellent, it is exceptional for the fetus to suffer mortality or serious morbidity within next 48 hours if not for even longer period unless something acute happens. For example, for NST this rate is 3.2 per 1000 and for CST it is as low as 0.4 per 1000 (Arias, 1993).

So, from the above observation it may be concluded that *CTG is an excellent test for fetal "wellness" rather than of fetal illness.*

Based on above, as widely quoted, the main use of CTG during antenatal period can be put as—*to allow more women with high risk pregnancy to continue their pregnancy—to greater maturity, safer maturity, better inducability or until the spontaneous onset of labor.*

The findings of Wheble et al (1989) of their survey of consultant obstetric units of UK that 92 percent UK units consider CTG alone or in combination with other tests to be the most reliable method of detecting fetal distress before labor—speaks for the undeniable role of the CTG in antepartum monitoring. The situation has not changed even after 23 years.

This is further supported by the following earlier report by Oats et al (1987):

In their study the authors recognised approximately 32 percent cases of one particular antenatal population to be sufficiently 'at risk' to merit an antenatal CTG at some stage. Of these 8 percent were found to show reduced fetal reserve and 1 percent critical reserve. Further, it was found that the incidence of small for date babies rose from 8 percent with normal CTG to 11 percent with suspicious CTG and 30 percent with pathological CTG.

INTRANATAL CTG—CRITICAL APPRAISAL

It has been shown that even with the worst form of tracing only 50–60 percent of fetuses get acidotic (Beard et al, 1971; Konje and Taylor, 1998). On the top of it—the startling results of the Dublin trial (Mac Donald et al, 1985) on 12,964 patients, comparing the value of electronic FH monitoring with that of ordinary intermittent auscultation with or without FBS—make the position of intrapartum CTG even more questionable. Here is the summary of the result of the above study:

There were no significant difference in the rates of low Apgar score, need for resuscitation, the need for transfer to special care nursery, rates of stillbirth and that of neonatal death between the two groups—whereas electronic monitoring group had slightly higher rate of cesarean section and forceps delivery.

However, the other portion of the result of this study stands as major point in favour of electronic monitoring in that—the incidence of neonatal seizures and persistent abnormal neurological signs followed by survival were more than double in the intermittent auscultation group in comparison to CTG group—a fact which lends the conclusion that in this group, at least temporary neurological damage, would have occurred.

Here are the results from other studies, which also need careful consideration.

As regards perinatal death, higher rate in auscultation group as compared to electronic FHR monitoring group with/without scalp blood sampling has been reported by workers from Sheffield and Copenhagen (Thacker, 1987).

A unique follow-up study of infants who had "ominous" CTG tracing during labor was conducted by Holmqvist et al (1984) amongst the survivors of a neonatal intensive care unit at 2 years of age and this is what they found—while 75 percent babies (3 out of 4) with persistent major neurological handicap had "ominous" tracing, only 20–30 percent of those with mild or transient neurological problems had such a tracing. More importantly, none of those without neurological problems had any such grossly abnormal tracing.

Westgren et al (1984) from their study of preterm infant found "ominous" heart rate patterns during labor more often in the 6 infants who had cerebral palsy at 2 years of age or showed a moderate delay of psychomotor development.

Niswander et al (1984) attempted to correlate the intervention protocol for fetal distress by comparing outcomes in fetuses who did or did not have an operative intervention during a period of abnormal tracing. They found that a lack of appropriate intervention was associated with neonatal seizures though not with cerebral palsy. The observation of Painter et al (1988) also tends to support the above finding as they noted higher incidence of neurological abnormalities during the first year of life amongst children with abnormal FHR pattern—though long-term fixed neurological deficit was not observed in these children in their 6 to 9 years follow-up. Don't support the above findings of reversible, perhaps because of intervention, neurological abnormality in presence of abnormal tracing the use of electronic FHR monitoring as a means of identifying the need for intervention and also the proposition that the cases of grossly abnormal tracing should be taken seriously.

As regards, intermittent auscultation of FHR as a method of intrapartum fetal monitoring, though several studies (not all) have shown that it is as good as CTG monitoring specially in low risk cases, data from the collaborative perinatal project has shown that this method is unable to anticipate fetal jeopardy (Benson et al, 1968).

INTERMITTENT AUSCULTATION—
THE GROUND REALITY

"Despite ACOG's (American College of Obstetrics and Gynaecology) endorsement–intermittent auscultation of FH rate is rarely used in the United States and continous electronic monitoring remains firmly as the current standard of care" (Arias, 1993). Here is the more recent report—85% of births in USA get monitored by CTG (National Vital Statistics Report, USA, 2003).

Here are some of the reasons for this resistance on the part of the obstetrician (also see Chapter 17) to accept the ACOG's findings and recommendation.

a. *Relative shortage of labour room staff* to provide for the 1:1 nurse-to-patient ratio that is required for such manual monitoring procedure. Besides, such manpower provision would be *very expensive* to arrange and almost impossible to conform to.

b. Intermittent auscultation is not very practical specially when labor room is busy.

c. Lack of pointed studies evaluating the accuracy of this simple auscultation methodology (Arias, 1993).

d. Lack of adequate definition of the frequency and duration of auscultation in low-risk patients (Arias, 1993).

e. Low-risk patients are not 'no-risk' patients.

f. Intuitive conviction that intermittent auscultation is inaccurate and unreliable.

g. The feeling that a return to intermittent auscultation negates the knowledge acquired during the last 35 years about different types and degrees of FHR alterations during labor.

Hence, it is no wonder that not only in States but also in UK CTG is used almost universally (Carter and Steer, 1993). Here is to quote, in support of the above, the general agreement of the 'working party on cardiotocograph technology' of Royal College of Obstetricians and Gynaecologists of London who met in March, 1993 (Cater and Steer, 1993)—"Cardiotocography is here to stay for the foreseeable future". We are standing today at 20 years since but the same comments still holds good.

Actually, since there is no option to monitoring fetus in labor because of the proven potential for its facing hypoxic threat during this critical period and since intermittent auscultation is not a very practical and reliable method of monitoring fetus in labor, *CTG seem to stand out as a very simple, non-invasive (when external method is used), auditable, objective alternative offering even ambulatory and telemetric monitoring facility and even on-line computer analysis option of the emerging tracing.*

TWO INSUPERABLE PROBLEMS OF CTG MONITORING

I. Inability of CTG to differentiate the three stages of hypoxia namely:
- Transient hypoxemia without metabolic acidosis

- Persistent hypoxia with metabolic acidosis
- Hypoxia bad enough to cause brain damage or mortality.

II. Virtual uselessness of CTG in acute hypoxic episodes like abruption of placenta, cord prolapse, uterine scar rupture, etc.

CTG THROUGH THE EYES OF "MEDICAL ECONOMISTS"

Finally let us look at CTG monitoring through the eyes of a 'medical economist' i.e. from the angle of 'return on investment' or trade off. No doubt from such purely business angle and statistical angle fetal monitoring by CTG (even by FBS and pH estimation which is a far more reliable test) may not be a very profitable activity because of (naturally) very low incidence of the related fetal and neonatal disasters. For example, despite the reported incidence of acidosis (pH less than 7.20) of 12 percent to 20 percent at birth the incidence of cerebral palsy is only approximately 2 per 1000 (Arias, 1993) and the incidence of intrapartum fetal death at term in the absence of risk factors is less than 1 per 25,000 patients—according to the report of Collaborative perinatal study (Lilien, 1970). But in medicine isn't often the case? For example everyday millions of routine EGG and chest X-ray being done to detect a meager few abnormality, everyday so many unnecessary surgeries being done for inconsequential lesions due to use of ultrasonography.

The problem with fetal monitoring is—*who can attach a value to a life or an undamaged brain.* To quote professor RW Beard of St Mary's Medical school, London "The only way to resolve this is to ask woman how they regard such a trade off. Woman would much rather undergo an unnecessary cesarean section than risk giving birth to a brain-damaged child" (Beard, 1993).

Even when explained to the pregnant mothers (even those who have to pay heavily for the test)—that CTG monitoring gives 50 percent false positive result—they interpret the communication as—the test gives 50 percent good result (i.e. the other 50 percent which does not give false positive result—like the phrase—"glass is not half empty, it is half full") and, in absence of any easy, cheap and suitable alternative, they welcome CTG monitoring for their fetus (Debdas, 1997).

UNDISPUTED PLACE

Let us conclude by listing the more or less undisputed indications of use of CTG for monitoring fetus (also see Chapter 3—Scope of Use of Cardiotocography).

- High risk antenatal cases in order to take them to—higher maturity, safer maturity, better inducability or until spontaneous onset of labor.
- Diabetics
- Oligohydramnios
- Prolonged rupture of membranes (24 hours+)
- APH cases
- Multiple pregnancy
- Induction of labor at least once when the painful contraction starts. This, in effect, is a sort of 'Contraction stress test' (CST)
- As 'Admission test' for all unbooked cases entering spontaneous labor
- Maternal pyrexia in labor
- Meconium stained liquor specially fresh meconium
- For confirming the diagnosis of premature labor (by definition there has to be 'documented' uterine contraction of the frequency of 4/20 minutes or 8/60 minutes to label a case as one of premature labor)
- For titrating the dose of tocolytic
- For cases of diminished DFMC
- For all patients who are getting continuous Epidural analgesia in labor
- In the cases of slow labor (uterine inertia) to find out whether it is, of hypotonic or hypertonic type so as to be able to manage the case appropriately. This requires internal tocometry

- If one wants to use oxytocin drip in a grande multipara or in a case of post-cesarean pregnancy, one must use CTG. Here also internal tocometry is required to titrate the dose of oxytocin
- For all mothers who electively want such sophisticated monitoring for their fetus.

FURTHER READING

1. Arias F. Practical Guide to High Risk Pregnancy and Delivery, 2nd edn, St Louis: Mosby year book. 1993;3–20, 301–18, 413–29.
2. Beard RW, Filshie GM, Knight CA, Roberts GM. J Obstet Gynaecol, Br Commonwealth. 1971;78:865–81.
3. Beard RW. Department of Obstetrics and Gynaecology, St Mary's Hospital Medical School, London: "The Obstetricians dilemma"—written for the Department of Health, NHS, UK (Personal communication), 1993.
4. Benson RC, Shubeck F, Deutschberger, et al. Obstet Gynecol 1968;32:259
5. Carter MC, Steer PJ. Brit J Obstet Gynaecol 1993;100(Supple 9):1–36.
6. D'Souza R, Arulkumaran S. 'Intrapartum fetal surveillance' in the book Best Practice in Labor and Delivery, Edited by Warren R Arulkumaran S, 2009;38–53.
7. Edwin C, Arulkumaran S. Electronic fetal heart monitoring in current & future practice. The Journal of O & G of India, 2008; 58: 121–30.
8. FIGO News: Guidelines for the use of fetal monitoring. Int J Gynecol Obstet 1987;25:159–67.
9. Holmqvist P, Svenningsen NW, Ingemarsson I. Acta Obstet Gynecol Scand 1984;63:527–32.
10. Konje JC Taylor DJ. Objective Structured Clinical Examination in Obstetrics & Gynaecology, Oxford Blackwell Science, 1998:103.
11. Lilian AA. Am J Obstet Gynecol 1970;107:595.
12. Low JA, Me Grath MJ, Marshall SJ, Fischer-Fay A, Karchmar EJ. Am J Obstet Gynecol 1986;154:769–76.
13. Mac Donald D, Grant A, Sheridan-Pereira M, et al. Am J Obstet Gynecol 1985;152:524–39.
14. Niswander K, Henson G, Elbourne D, et al. Lancet 1984;2:827–31.

15. Nordstrom L, Ingemarsson I, Kublickas M, Persson B, Shimojo N, Westgren M. Brit J Obstet Gynaecol 1995;102:894–99.

16. Oats JN, Chew FTK, Rarren VJ. Aust NZ Obstet Gynaecol 1987;27:82–86.

17. Painter MJ, Scott M, Hirsch RP, O'Donoghue P, Depp R. Am J Obstet Gynecol 1988;159:854–58.

18. Thacker SB. Am J Obstet Gynecol 1987;156:24–30.

19. Westgren M, Holmqvist P, Ingemarsson I, Svenningsen NW. Obstet Gynecol 1984;63:355–59.

20. Wheble AM, Gillimer MDG, Spencer JAD, Sykes GS. Brit J Obstet Gynaecol 1989;96:1140–7.

21. William's Obstetrics, 23rd edition, Edited by Cunningham FG, Leveno KJ, Bloom SL, Hauth JC, Rouse DJ, Spong CY, Intrapartum Assessment,Mc Graw Hill, New York, 2010;410–3

Special Features of CTG of Second Stage of Labor

With second stage CTG one starts with a handicap or minus because – *Decelerations—a notorious sign of fetal distress—are virtually ever present in second stage of labor.*

Technical Problems of CTG Monitoring in Second Stage of Labor

- Transducer displacement—FH monitoring by external mode is difficult in second stage because the abdominal transducer often gets displaced due to—uncontrollable, excessive body movement by the mother, due to her pushing efforts and due to associated irregular excessive breathing.
- Breath-holding during pushing—This being the rule, it invariably brings in varying degree of recurrent additional stress on gas-exchange by the fetus making assessment difficult.

Physiological Physical Problems of Second Stage

- Invariable occurrence head compression – This is occasioned by the natural resistance offered by the lower vagina and perineum—which is high and prolonged in primi—causing stimulation of vagal center and reflex deceleration.
- Even cord compression due to the above tight coursing through the birth canal have been implicated for decelerations and bradycardia (Cunningham et al, 2010).

Trace Interpretation Problems of Second Stage

- The above two physiological response causes major confusion in interpretation as to how to label these decelerations—Non-Hypoxic or Hypoxic.
- Since in most cases contractions come in very quick succession specially towards the end—it is sometimes difficult to assess the baseline character of the tracing.
- While some authors reported 33 percent incidence of 'variable deceleration' some others reported 36 percent incidence of 'unclassified pattern/non-reassuring' pattern. (Stone and Murray, 1995).

The overall conclusion the review of literature would tend to offer is the unpredictability of FHR tracings in second stage.

Ominous Features in Second Stage Tracing

- Sustained bradycardia below 90 bpm.
- Progressive bradycardia with each bearing down effort.
- Loss of baseline variability.
- Failure of the fetal heart rate, to recover completely in-between contractions.

Occurrence of these should call for assisted delivery.

FURTHER READING

1. Cunningham FG, Leveno KJ, Bloom SL, Hauth JC, Rouse DJ and Spong CY: Intrapartum Assessment, in William's Obstetrics: 23rd edition, Mc Graw Hill, New York, 2010;425.

2. Ingemarsson I, Arulkumaran S, Ingemarsson E, Tambyraja RI, Ratnam SS. Obstet Gynecol 1986;68:800–06.

3. Ingemarsson I, Ingemarsson E and Spencer JAD. Fetal Heart Rate Monitoring—A Practical Guide. Oxford: Oxford University Press, 1993;41.

4. Stone PR, Murray HG. John Bonnar (Ed). Recent Advances in Obst and Gynae, vol-19, London: Churchill Livingstone, 1995;19:45–62.

NICE Guidelines for CTG Interpretation

National Institute of Clinical Excellence (NICE) has prepared the following guidelines for interpretation of CTG traces (September, 2007) which is really not different from other guidelines that can be found in the literature.

In this system, like other systems, only the following *four features* has to be studied in any trace :

  I. Baseline FHR (bpm)
  II. Baseline variability of FHR (bpm)
 III. Decelerations
 IV. Accelerations

Classification of CTG Traces on the Basis of the Gravity of the Above Four CTG Features

Normal / Reassuring Trace

Baseline FHR	110–160 bpm
Baseline variability	>/= 5 bpm
Decelerations	None
Accelerations	Present – 15/15

Non-Reassuring Trace

Baseline FHR	• On low side—100–109
	• On high side—161–180

Baseline variability of FHR	<5 for 40–90 minutes
Deceleration	• Typical Variable Deceleration with over 50% of contractions occurring over 90 minutes
	• Single prolonged deceleration for up to 3 minutes
Accelerations	Absence of accelerations with otherwise normal trace is of uncertain significance

Abnormal Trace

Baseline FHR	• On low side—<100 bpm
	• On high side—>180 bpm
Baseline variability	<5 for 90 minutes
Decelerations	Either –
	• Atypical variable decelerations with over 50% of contractions or
	• Late decelerations - *both for 30 minutes* or
	• Single prolonged deceleration for more than 3 minutes
Acceleration	None

No doubt it is a simple guideline but in practice so many mixed types of traces are seen increasing the bulk of 'intermediate' or '*suspicious*' type of tracing and consequent obstetrician's distress and high cesarean section (CS) rate—*four fold* if CTG alone is used to diagnose fetal distress (Magowan, Owen and Drife, 2009).

And not only this, misinterpretation and consequent fetal and neonatal problem also keep happening leading to law suit in spite of the guidelines. NICE guideline has been there since 2001.

Finally, "It is indefensible not to take action" on Suspicious and Pathological Traces (D'Souza and Arulkumaran, 2009).

FURTHER READING

1. Magowan B, Owen P, Drife J: Clinical Obst Gynae, 2nd edition, Monitoring the Fetus in Labor, Elsevier, Edinburgh, 2009; pp. 331-43.
2. NICE (National Institute for Clinical Excellence) Guideline :The use of Electronic fetal monitoring: the use and interpretation of Cardiotocography in Intrapartum Fetal Surveillance, 2001, London.
3. NICE (National Institute for Clinical Excellence) Guideline :The Clinical Guideline No. 55, Induction of labour, RCOG press, September 2007, London

CTG, BPP and Doppler—Comparative Scope and Inter-relation

SCIENTIFIC PHILOSOPHY OF USING THE ABOVE THREE METHODS

Doppler

This investigation tells us the fetal 'climate' that has been during last *few weeks to a month* and also what it is possibly going to be over the same time period. It is somewhat comparable to the value of HbA1C for a diabetic patient during past may be two moths or so.

BPP—Biophysical Profile

This investigation tells us the fetal 'weather' that has been and is going to be during the last and also the coming few days—whether it has been or going to be sunny or cloudy or rainy etc.

CTG

This tells us the condition of fetal aerosphere for the next 2–6 hours or a bit longer. This is analogous to the current or random blood sugar level of a diabetic patient.

COMPARATIVE SCOPE OF USE OF THE ABOVE METHODS IN RELATION TO THE STATE OF PREGNANCY—WHETHER ANTENATAL OR INTRANATAL

For Fetal Monitoring during Antenatal Period

All the above three methods are applicable. However, CTG is usually primarily employed because of the ease of its applicability and low skill and cost involved. BPP and Doppler are employed in selected cases usually only for chronic fetal affection cases.

For Fetal Monitoring during Intrapartum Period

Only CTG is applicable at this rather acute period because it is only this technology that can *monitor the stressor,* i.e. the uterine contraction which invariably stresses placental circulation and through that the fetal homeostasis.

The other two methods are not designed for it and hence unsuitable for intrapartum monitoring. Besides this, these methods cannot be used for the long period that needs to be covered for intrapartum monitoring, i.e. a duration of 10–12 hours of labor and also cannot be done repeatedly for continuous cover. Moreover, in contrast to CTG machine, it is not a standard labor room equipment.

COMPARATIVE CLINICAL INDICATION OF USE OF THESE METHODS

- For cases of *chronic fetal affection,* e.g. Growth restriction cases and cases where disease process is slow and damage occurs insidiously, e.g. chronic hypertension, chronic renal disease, diabetes, SLE cases
  - BPP and Doppler are indicated and very useful here
- For acute assessment and acute-on-chronic assessment of fetus as in labor
  - CTG is indicated.

This may be combined with F-ECG and Fetal blood sampling and pH estimation where required.

WHERE BPP AND DOPPLER END—CTG BEGINS

If fetal assessment by any or both BPP and Doppler show abnormal result and circumstances—clinical (too premature) and facilitywise (infrastructure and specialist cover) are not very conducive to immediate delivery some hours—may be few days—can be gained by doing continuous CTG provided CTG remains normal.

CONCLUSION

The above three tests are complementary and have their indispensable place.

FURTHER READING

William's Obstetrics: 23rd edition, Edited by Cunningham FG, Leveno KJ, Bloom SL, Hauth JC, Rouse DJ and Spong CY, Intrapartum Assessment, Mc Graw Hill, New York, 2010. pp. 410-43.

36

CTG and Fetal Acidosis

Unfortunately, the correlation is quite poor as can be seen in the following references.

ABNORMAL FHR TRACING→TO→ACIDOSIS INTERVAL

Fleischer et al (1982), demonstrated that with an averagely grown fetus at term with clear amniotic fluid, 50% of fetuses took the following time duration to become acidiotic after an abnormal or suspicious trace:

With repeated late decelerations	–	115 min (2 hours)
With repeated variable deceleration	–	145 min (2 1/2 hours)
With flat trace (baseline variability of less than 5 bpm)	–	185 min (3 hours)

Here are two often quoted reference on the above -

Even with the worst pattern of tracing only 50–60 percent of fetuses were found to be Acidotic (Beard, 1971; Konje and Taylor, 1998).

CORRELATION BETWEEN CTG FINDING AND SCALP pH VALUE

The cut-off value for normalcy of scalp pH is generally taken as 7.20

CTG Excellent (i.e. its all four parameters are normal)	–	Risk of pH being less than 7.20 is—only 2%.
CTG Non-reassuring	–	Risk of pH being less than 7.20 is—only 20%.
CTG Abnormal	–	Risk of pH being less than 7.20 is—only 50%.

FURTHER READING

1. Beard RW, Filshie GM et al. Significance of the changes in the continuous fetal heart rate in the first stage of labour, J Obstet Gynaecol Brit Cwlth, 1971;78:865–81.
2. Fleischer A, Schulman H, Jagani N, Mitchell J, Randolph G. Am J Obstet Gynecol 1982;144:55–60.
3. Konje JC and Taylor DJ: Objective Structured Clinical Examination in Obstetrics & Gynaecology,Oxford Blackwell Science, 1998:103.
4. Magowan B, Owen P, Drife J: Clinical Obst Gynae, 2nd edition, Monitoring the fetus in labor, Elsevier, Edinburgh, 2009;331–43

CTG and Cerebral Palsy

The questions here are two:
1. Whether intrapartum hypoxic injury usually cause cerebral palsy?
2. Whether it is preventable by doing intranatal CTG monitoring for diagnosing hypoxia early and arrange to deliver the fetus before brain damage has taken place?

FETAL HEART RATE PATTERNS AND BRAIN DAMAGE

Here is to quote some studies on this issue –

- No specific pattern of trace could be correlated with neurological injury (Rosen and Dickinson, 1992).
- On retrospective study of CTG traces of the neurologically impaired children, in 70% cases persistant Non-reactive tracing was found right on admission in labor suggesting thereby that injury would have occurred prior to arrival to hospital (Phelan and Ahn, 1994)
- On retrospective review of CTG tracing of neonates with neurological impairment, in 75% of cases the condition was found to be non-preventable by their CTG character (Phelan et al, 1996).
- Review of World literature published between 1966 and 2006 found no benefit of FHR monitoring by CTG in prevention of perinatal brain injury (Graham et al, 2006).

CRITERIA NECESSARY TO CONSIDER BIRTH ASPHYXIA AS A CAUSE OF CEREBRAL PALSY (ACOG, 2006B)

- Evidence of metabolic acidosis has to be present in cord blood
- There has to be occurrence of Hypoxic Ischemic Encephalopathy (HIE) of early onset and of moderate or severe degree
- The infant should have spastic quadriplagia and less commonly dyskinetic problem.

(Unilateral brain lesions are not a result of intrapartum hypoxia).

CONCLUSION

Obviously, the clinical correlation is poor but we will have to wait for results of further more sophisticated research before we can conclude and also hope for emergence of more pointed test.

FURTHER READING

1. Graham EM, Petersen SM, Christo DK et al: Intrapartum electronic fetal heart monitoring and the prevention of perinatal birth injury, Obstet Gynecol 2006;108:656.
2. Phelan JP, Ahn MO : Perinatal observations in 48 neurologically term infants, Am J Obstet Gynecol, 1994;171:424.
3. Phelan JP, Ahn MO, Korst L et al: Is intrapartum fetal brain injury in the term fetus preventable, Am J Obstet Gynecol, 1996;174:318.
4. Rosen MG, Dickinson JC: The incidence of cerebral palsy, Am J Obstet Gynecol, 1992;167:417.

Assumptions and Presumptions about CTG Monitoring

- Fetal distress is a slowly developing phenomenon
- So, CTG can make possible early detection of the compromised fetus when pathology was still in developing stage
- All fetal damage occurs only after the patient gets admitted in Hospital
  So close and constant monitoring right from admission by CTG should detect it and make it's salvage possible
- In contrast to the above assumption, lot of evidence have accumulated over last 20 years which proves that most damaged fetuses suffered their insults before arrival at labor units
- If a dead or damaged baby is delivered and if it was being monitored by CTG then that CTG *tracing strip must provide some clue* that some detectable untoward thing had been happening
- *Finally, that*—**ALL dead and damaged fetuses were preventable.**

Review of world literature published between 1966 and 2006 found no benefit of FHR monitoring by CTG in prevention of perinatal brain injury (Graham et al, 2006).

Obviously, from a little instrument – a simple cardiac rate meter (rate recording device)-holding such great expectation is really unreasonable. However, wide publicity of such inflated expectations keeps fueling the fire of disappointment leading to often baseless litigation by the aggrieved couple.

[Also read the Chapter No. 37 – 'CTG and Cerebral Palsy']

FURTHER READING

1. Graham EM, Petersen SM, Christo DK, et al. Intrapartum electronic fetal heart monitoring and the prevention of perinatal birth injury, Obstet Gynecol 2006; 108:656.

2. William's Obstetrics: 23rd edition, edited by Cunningham FG, Leveno KJ, Bloom SL, Hauth JC, Rouse DJ and Spong CY, Intrapartum Assessment, Mc Graw Hill, New York 2010; 410–43.

Training and Education for CTG Interpretation

Its need cannot be over emphasized since there is so much inter and also intra observer variability in this vital issue as described in several chapters in this book.

WHO SHOULD BE TRAINED?

- All obstetrics resident doctors including House Surgeon and Registrars
- Midwives and all Nurses posted in Obstetric wards and labor room.

Category of training	COMPULSORY
Frequency of training	Every six months
Duration of training	Half day (3 hours)
Duty status of the trainee	On official study leave, i.e. off from clinical work and on call duty
On the job training	Monthly departmental case review
New recruitments	Two hours introductory training in the department
Availability of Study Material	Books and CDs should be available in the department

eFM - RCOG

RCOG & RCM have jointly prepared a good 'interactive' electronic CTG training module called *eFM* in which one can take self examination. Pass mark is 70%.

One is able to access the resource for a fee of £100 per annum.

FURTHER READING

1. D'Souza R and Arulkumaran S: 'Intrapartum Fetal Surveillance' in the book Best Practice in Labor and Delivery, Edited by Warren R and Arulkumaran S, 2009;38–53.
2. RCOG – type in google Search - eLfH , eFM for details.

CTG—Complications and Contraindications

EXTERNAL METHOD

CTG done by *External Method* is a very safe procedure. The only risk is that of current leakage which can be avoided by the following precautions:

- The patient's cable must be so positioned that it should not come into contact with any other electrical equipment or with the metal bed-frame.
- Transducer gel, electrode gel or any other wet substance should not be kept on the monitor.
- Three pin plug with good earthing facility is mandatory.
- The machine should not be used in presence of inflammable anesthetics.

INTERNAL METHOD

CTG done by *Internal Method* is also generally quite safe.

However, the following types of fetal and maternal injuries have been reported:

Due to Malapplication of Electrode of the Fetus

Local injury due to electrode being pulled off and small bleeding and localised infection as a result. In breech, it must not be applied on the Scrotum.

Due to Malapplication of Intrauterine Catheter

This is a real risk though does not happen commonly when done by an experienced person. Possible risks are –

- Penetration of placenta specially when it is posterior and low
- Uterine perforation
- Injury to fetal vessel and fetal bleeding
- Cord complication due to its entanglement with intra-uterine catheter
- Spurious recording by the intra-uterine pressure catheter—due to its blockage by vernix etc, catheter tip lying in a dry place within the uterus—leading to inappropriate management of the case.
- Puerperal sepsis.

CONTRAINDICATIONS TO DOING CTG

CTG by internal method is contraindicated in presence of the following maternal infective diseases:

HIV, HSV, Hepatitis B and Hepatitis C.

FURTHER READING

1. American Academy of Pediatrics and American College of Obstetricians & Gynecologists: Intrapartum and Postpartum care of the mother. In Guidelines of Perinatal care, 6th ed, Washington DC, 2007;146.
2. William's Obstetrics: 23rd edition, Edited by Cunningham FG, Leveno KJ, Bloom SL, Hauth JC, Rouse DJ and Spong CY, Intrapartum Assessment, Mc Graw Hill, New York, 2010;410–43.

Index